Plant based weight loss cookbook for seniors

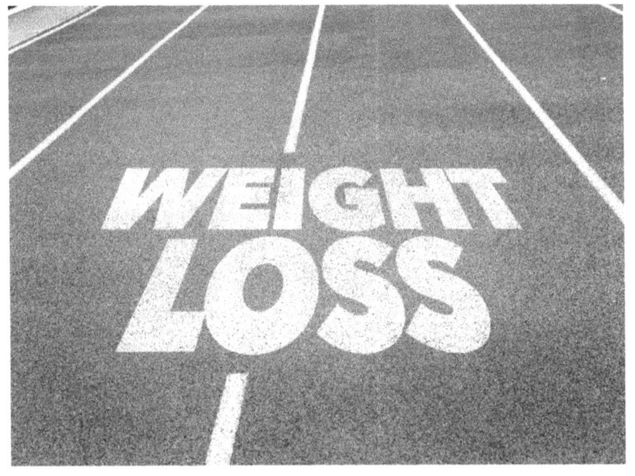

Discover Healthier Living with Our Delicious Recipes for a Vibrant Lifestyle.

Elba R. Norman

1

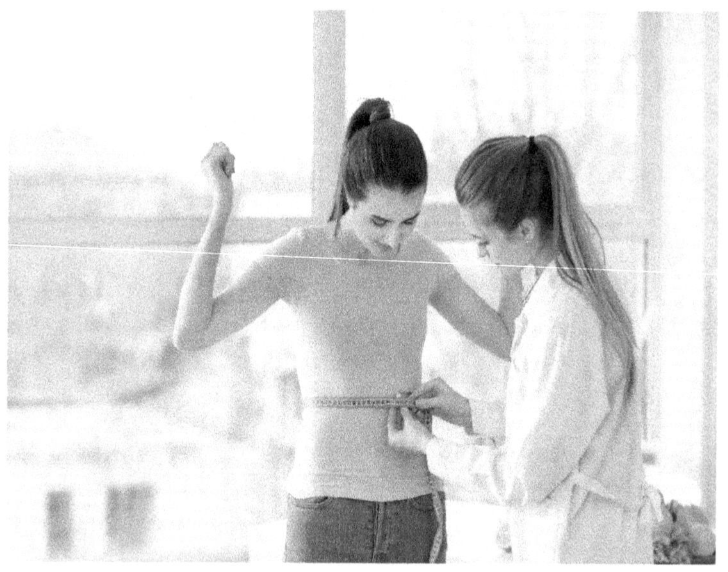

Table of contents

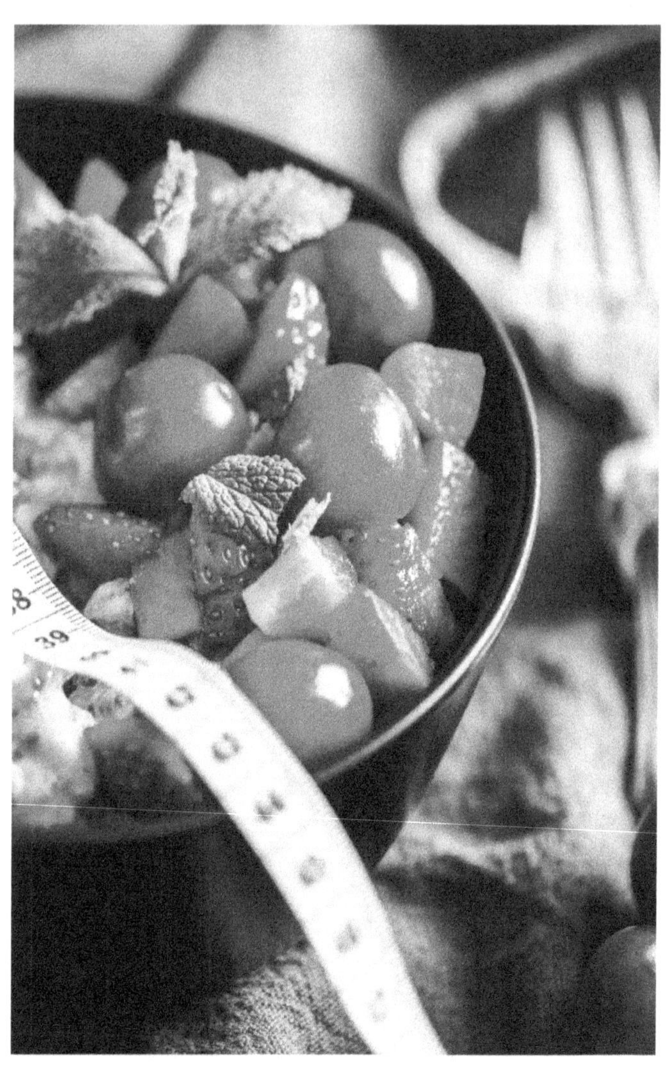

INTRODUCTION

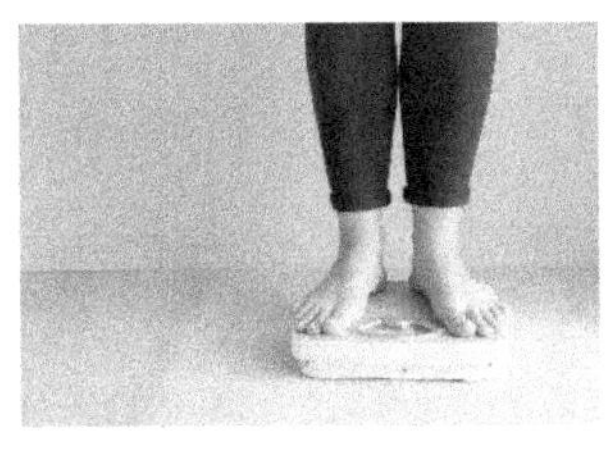 Nathan's senior-year journey toward a healthy living began with an insight that went beyond the accepted conventions of aging. Nathan found himself dealing with the aftereffects of a sedentary lifestyle and the inevitable extra pounds that came with it as he entered his golden years. He began on a transforming trip, inspired by the pages of a plant-based weight loss cookbook expressly intended for seniors, determined to break free from the shackles of lethargy and excess weight.

Nathan's life was turned upside down when he faced the harsh reality of his condition at a routine doctor's visit. Recognizing the hazards connected with age-related weight gain, his doctor proposed a more holistic approach to wellbeing. Nathan came across the plant-based weight loss recipe that would become his compass on this fresh path.

Nathan was initially drawn to the cookbook because of its vivid appearance and promises of regeneration. He excitedly dug into its pages, enthralled by the idea of reducing unwanted pounds through the power of plant-based nourishment. What emerged was not just a collection of recipes, but a comprehensive handbook customized to the special requirements and challenges confronting elders seeking to recapture their vitality.

With the publication of the cookbook, Nathan was given a road map to learning the core concepts of plant-based diet. It emphasized the importance of a diet rich in fruits, vegetables, whole grains, and legumes in aiding weight loss, increasing energy levels, and improving general well-being. Nathan felt empowered and optimistic as he read through the first few pages, learning that age was not a barrier to adopting healthy behaviors.

Nathan began experimenting with the cookbook's vast assortment of recipes, armed with newfound information. From robust salads to flavorful plant-based stews, each item was meticulously designed to provide the ideal mix of nutrients for seniors. The dishes in the cookbook not only focused on weight loss, but also on bone health, heart function, and cognitive well-being, addressing the complex demands of people in their golden years.

Nathan's kitchen turned traditional views about senior meals into a celebration of colorful, plant-based cuisine, transforming it into a laboratory of flavors and wellbeing. The perfume of herbs and spices floated through his house, creating a welcoming environment that mirrored the wonderful changes taking place within his body.

However, the journey was not without its difficulties. Nathan had doubts and cravings for classic comfort foods, but the cookbook was a constant friend, offering alternatives and support. He noted a slow but substantial improvement in his energy levels, weight, and overall health over time.

Nathan's tale exemplifies the transforming impact of adopting a plant-based diet in one's golden years. His experience with the senior weight reduction cookbook is a light of hope for others navigating the obstacles of aging. As he continues to enjoy the bounty of life, Nathan serves as a living example of how it's never too late to begin a journey toward a healthier, more vibrant self.

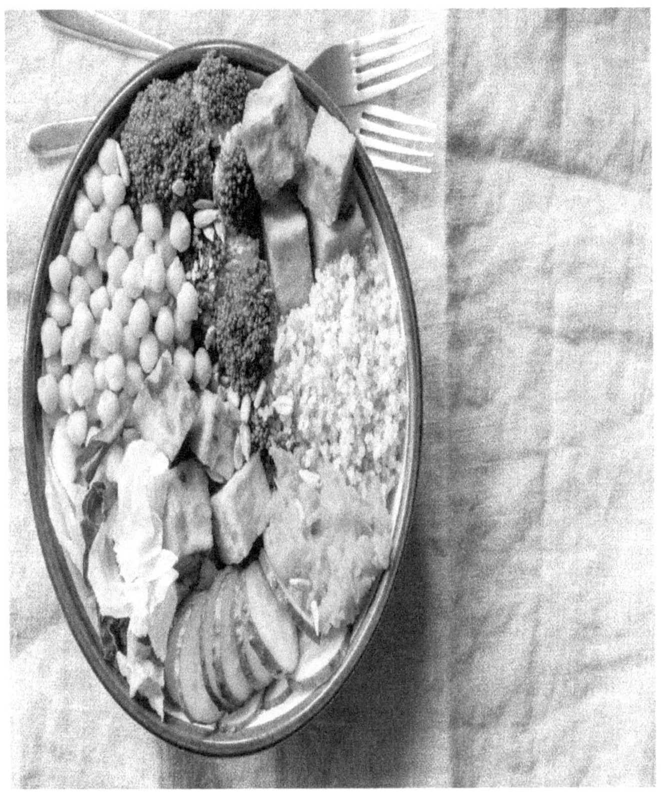

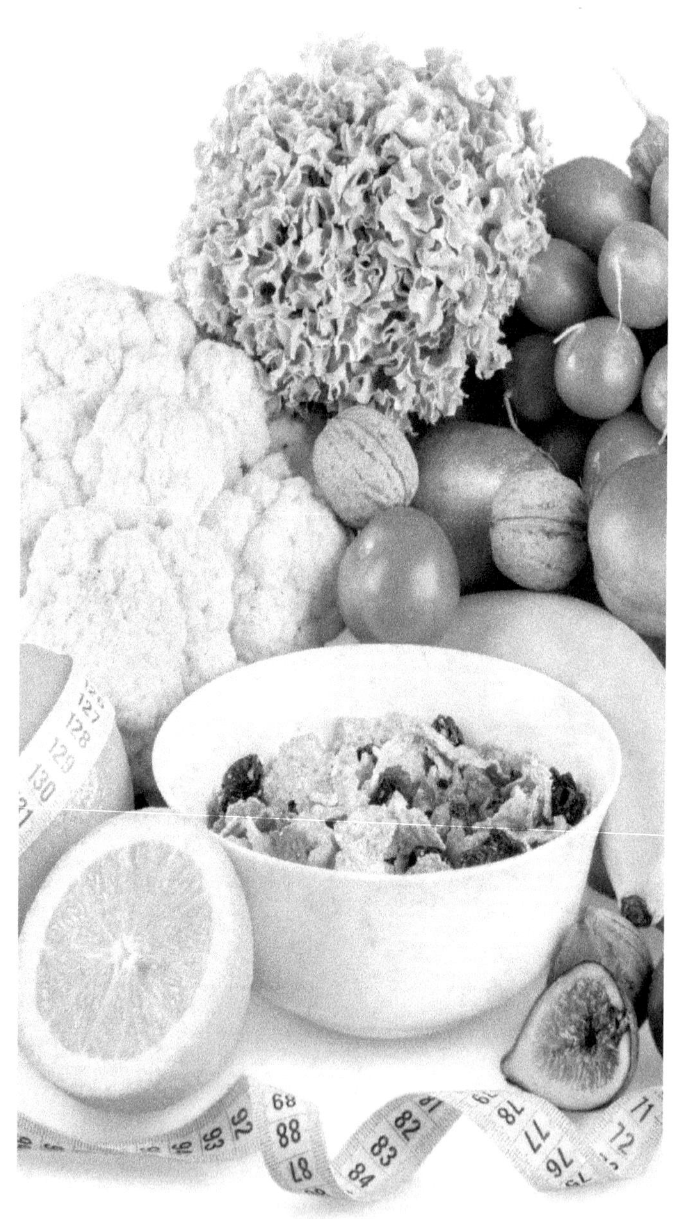

CHAPTER 1: BREAKFAST TO START YOUR DAY

Quinoa Breakfast Bowl

Ingredients

- 1 cup quinoa, rinsed
- 2 cups almond milk (or any milk of your choice)
- 1 tablespoon honey or maple syrup
- 1 teaspoon vanilla extract
- 1/2 teaspoon cinnamon
- Pinch of salt
- 1 cup mixed berries (strawberries, blueberries, raspberries)
- 1 banana, sliced
- 1/4 cup chopped nuts (such as almonds, walnuts, or pecans)
- 2 tablespoons chia seeds
- Greek yogurt for topping (optional)

Instructions:

1. Rinse Quinoa: To remove any bitter taste, rinse the quinoa under cold water.

2. Quinoa: Combine the rinsed quinoa, almond milk, honey or maple syrup, vanilla essence, cinnamon, and a bit of salt in a medium pot. Bring to a boil, then lower to a low heat, cover, and cook for 15-20 minutes, or until the quinoa is tender and the liquid has been absorbed. With a fork, fluff the quinoa.

3. Toppings: Prepare your toppings while the quinoa is cooking. Wash the berries and cut the banana into slices.

4. Assemble Bowls: When the quinoa has finished cooking, divide it among serving bowls. Arrange the quinoa on top of the sliced banana, mixed berries, and chopped nuts.

5. Chia Seeds: For an added burst of nourishment and a delicious texture, sprinkle chia seeds over the bowls.

6. Optional Greek Yogurt: For smoothness and extra protein, top with a dollop of Greek yogurt.

7. If preferred, drizzle with honey or maple syrup before serving. Warm quinoa breakfast bowls are a wholesome and tasty way to start the day!

Chia Seed Pudding

Ingredients:

- 1/4 cup chia seeds
- 1 cup milk (you can use almond milk, coconut milk, or any milk of your choice)
- 1-2 tablespoons sweetener (such as honey, maple syrup, or agave nectar)
- 1/2 teaspoon vanilla extract

- Optional toppings: fresh fruits, nuts, seeds, or granola

Instructions:

1. Chia Seeds with Milk: Combine the chia seeds and milk in a bowl. Stir thoroughly to ensure that the chia seeds are uniformly dispersed throughout the milk.

2. Sweetener and Vanilla: To the chia seed mixture, add the sweetener of your choice (honey, maple syrup, or agave nectar) and vanilla essence. Stir one more to combine these ingredients.

3. Allow to set: Wrap the bowl in plastic wrap or store it in an airtight container. Allow at least 2 hours, ideally overnight, for the mixture to solidify in the refrigerator. The chia seeds will absorb the liquid and form a pudding-like texture.

4. Stir Once More: After the first setting time, give the pudding another vigorous stir to break up any clumps and guarantee a smooth texture. If the pudding is too thick, add a little more milk to achieve the required consistency.

5. Spoon the chia seed pudding into serving bowls or jars to serve. For extra taste and texture, cover it with fresh fruits, nuts, seeds, or granola.

Avocado Toast with Tomato

Ingredients:

- 2 slices of your favorite bread (sourdough, whole grain, or multigrain work well)
- 1 ripe avocado
- 1 medium-sized tomato, sliced
- 1 tablespoon olive oil

- Salt and pepper to taste
- Optional toppings: red pepper flakes, lemon juice, feta cheese, or a poached egg.

Instructions:

1. Toasted bread: Toast the bread slices to your preferred crispiness. A toaster or a toaster oven can be used.

2. Make the Avocado: Cut the ripe avocado in half and remove the pit while the bread is browning. Scoop out the avocado flesh and place it in a bowl.

3. Avocado, mashed: Mash the avocado with a fork until it reaches the desired amount of creaminess. If you prefer a chunkier texture, mash it less; if you prefer a smoother texture, mash it more.

4. Season the avocado as follows: Season with salt and pepper to taste. Add a

splash of lemon juice for added flavor and to keep the avocado from browning.

5. Prepare the Toast: Once the bread has been toasted, evenly sprinkle the mashed avocado on each piece.

6. Sliced Tomatoes: On top of the mashed avocado, arrange the tomato slices. Arrange them evenly across the surface.

7. Drizzle with extra virgin olive oil: A tablespoon of olive oil should be drizzled over the tomato slices. This brings the flavors together and creates a rich flavor.

8. Optional Extras: Sprinkle with red pepper flakes for added heat, crumble feta cheese for extra creaminess, or top with a poached egg for protein.

9. Season once more (optional): For more taste, sprinkle a touch of salt and pepper on top of the tomatoes or any other toppings.

10. Serve and have fun: Your Avocado Toast with Tomato is now ready to eat! Serve immediately and enjoy the creamy avocado, juicy tomatoes, and crunchy toast.

Sweet Potato and Spinach Hash

Ingredients:

- 2 medium-sized sweet potatoes, peeled and diced into small cubes
- 2 cups fresh spinach, chopped
- 1 onion, finely chopped
- 2 cloves garlic, minced
- 1 red bell pepper, diced
- 1 teaspoon smoked paprika
- 1/2 teaspoon cumin
- Salt and pepper to taste
- 2 tablespoons olive oil
- 4 large eggs (optional, for serving)

- Fresh parsley, chopped (for garnish)

Instructions:

1. Prepare the sweet potatoes as follows: Peel and cut the sweet potatoes into small, uniform pieces.

2. Cook the Vegetables: Warm the olive oil in a large skillet over medium heat. Sauté the chopped onions and minced garlic until softened.

3. Cook the sweet potatoes as follows: To the skillet, add the diced sweet potatoes. Cook until the sweet potatoes are soft and gently caramelized, stirring occasionally. This should take between 10 and 12 minutes.

4. Combine the bell pepper and spinach: Cook for a another 3-4 minutes, or until the red bell pepper is cooked, in the skillet.

Cook until the spinach is wilted, stirring frequently.

5. Season the Hash with: Sprinkle the mixture with smoked paprika, cumin, salt, and pepper. Stir well to coat the vegetables evenly with the spices.

6. Finish the cooking: Continue cooking for another 2-3 minutes to enable the flavors to mingle.

7. Eggs poached or fried: Poach or fry eggs in a separate pan according to your desire.

8. Serve: Serve the sweet potato and spinach hash on individual dishes.

   If preferred, top each plate with a poached or fried egg.

   Garnish with chopped fresh parsley.

Berry banana smoothie Bowl

Ingredients:

- 1 frozen banana, sliced
- 1 cup mixed berries (strawberries, blueberries, raspberries)
- 1/2 cup plain Greek yogurt
- 1/4 cup almond milk (or any milk of your choice)
- 1 tablespoon honey (optional, for sweetness)
- 1/4 cup granola
- 1 tablespoon chia seeds
- Fresh fruits (sliced banana, berries) for topping
- Coconut flakes and mint leaves for garnish (optional)

Introduction:

1. Preparation of the Frozen Fruit: Place the banana in the freezer for at least a few hours, if not overnight.

2. Make the Smoothie: Blend together the frozen banana slices, mixed berries,

Greek yogurt, almond milk, and honey (if using) in a blender.

Blend until the mixture is smooth and creamy. If the mixture is too thick, add a little more almond milk to get the correct consistency.

3. Pour into a mixing bowl: Fill a bowl halfway with the smoothie.

   Toppings are optional.

   Sprinkle the granola and chia seeds on top of the smoothie.

4. Fresh Fruits on top: Top with more fresh fruit pieces, such as banana slices and berries.

5. Optional garnish: For a refreshing touch, garnish with coconut flakes and mint leaves.

6. Serve right away: Enjoy the Berry Banana Smoothie Bowl right away while it's still cool and fresh.

7. Customize: Feel free to add other toppings to your smoothie bowl, such as almonds, seeds, or a dab of nut butter.

Oatmeal with Nut Butter

Ingredients:

- 1/2 cup old-fashioned rolled oats
- 1 cup milk (dairy or plant-based)
- 1 tablespoon nut butter (peanut butter, almond butter, or any nut butter of your choice)
- 1 banana, sliced
- 1 tablespoon honey or maple syrup (optional, for sweetness)
- 1/2 teaspoon vanilla extract
- Pinch of salt
- Toppings: sliced bananas, a drizzle of nut butter, chopped nuts (almonds,

walnuts, or pecans), and a sprinkle of cinnamon

Instructions

1. Make the Oatmeal: Combine the rolled oats, milk, vanilla extract, and a bit of salt in a saucepan.
   Over medium heat, bring the mixture to a simmer, stirring occasionally.

2. Stir and Simmer: Reduce the heat to low and continue to cook the oats until they reach the desired consistency, about 5-7 minutes.

3. Include Nut Butter: When the oatmeal is done, toss in your favorite nut butter. Mix until the nut butter is all mixed and the oats is creamy.

4. Adjust the sweetness to taste: Sweeten the oatmeal with honey or maple syrup if desired. Depending on your taste, adjust the sweetness.

5. Serve: Fill a bowl halfway with nut butter oatmeal.

6. Top with banana slices and nuts: Top the oats with sliced bananas, more nut butter, and a sprinkle of chopped nuts.

7. Optional: Sprinkle with Cinnamon: Sprinkle a pinch of cinnamon on top of the oats for added taste.

8. Warmest Regards: Serve the Nut Butter Oatmeal while it's still warm. The creamy texture, nutty flavor, and sweetness combine to provide a hearty and filling breakfast.

Veggie Breakfast Burrito

Ingredients:

- 4 large whole wheat or spinach tortillas
- 1 tablespoon olive oil
- 1 small onion, finely chopped
- 1 bell pepper, diced (any color)

- 1 zucchini, diced

- 1 cup cherry tomatoes, halved

- 1 cup black beans, drained and rinsed

- 1 teaspoon ground cumin

- 1 teaspoon chili powder

- Salt and pepper to taste

- 6 large eggs, scrambled

- 1 cup shredded cheese (cheddar, Monterey Jack, or a blend)

- 1 avocado, sliced

- Fresh cilantro, chopped (for garnish)

- Salsa and Greek yogurt (optional, for serving)

Introduction

1. Preparation of the Vegetables: Warm the olive oil in a large skillet over medium heat. Cook until the onion has softened.

2. Prepare the Vegetables: To the skillet, add diced bell pepper and zucchini. Cook

for a few minutes, or until the vegetables are cooked but still crunchy.

3. Tomatoes and black beans are optional: Add the cherry tomatoes and black beans and mix well. Cook for another 2-3 minutes, or until the tomatoes have softened somewhat.

4. Season the vegetables as follows: Season the vegetable mixture with cumin, chili powder, salt, and pepper. Stir the spices into the vegetables thoroughly.

5. Make the scrambled eggs: Place the vegetables on one side of the griddle and the scrambled eggs on the other. Cook, stirring periodically, until the eggs are just set.

6. Melt the cheese in the following ways: In the skillet, combine the scrambled eggs and the cooked vegetables. Allow the shredded cheese to melt over the mixture.

7. Heat the Tortillas: To make the tortillas malleable, heat them on a dry pan or microwave according to package directions.

8. Make the Burritos: Fill each tortilla with the veggie and egg mixture. Serve with sliced avocado and chopped cilantro on top.

9. Roll and fold: Fold each tortilla in half and roll it up tightly to form a burrito.

10. Serve: Immediately serve the Veggie Breakfast Burritos. You can serve them with salsa and Greek yogurt on the side, if desired.

Mango Coconut Parfait

Ingredients:

- 2 ripe mangoes, peeled, pitted, and diced
- 1 cup Greek yogurt (or coconut yogurt for a dairy-free option)

- 1 cup coconut flakes, toasted

- 2 tablespoons honey or maple syrup

- 1 teaspoon vanilla extract

- 1 cup granola (homemade or store-bought)

- Fresh mint leaves for garnish (optional)

Instructions

1. Make the Mango: Ripe mangoes should be peeled, pitted, and diced into small cubes.

2. Coconut Flakes, Toasted: Toast the coconut flakes in a dry skillet over medium heat until golden brown. To avoid burning, be sure to stir often. This should just take 3-5 minutes. Place aside.

3. Make the Yogurt Sweeter: In a mixing dish, combine the Greek yogurt, honey or maple syrup, and vanilla extract. Stir until thoroughly blended.

4. Make the Parfait: Lay the ingredients in serving glasses or bowls as follows:

Begin with a tablespoon of the sweetened yogurt in the bottom of the bowl.

Top with a layer of sliced mango.

5. Sprinkle with toasted coconut flakes.

6. Spread granola on top.

7. Layers that should be repeated: Continue layering until you reach the top of the glass or bowl.

8. Toppings to finish: Finish with a final layer of sliced mango, toasted coconut, and a few mint leaves for decoration, if preferred.

9. Chill before serving: enable the Mango Coconut Parfait to chill for at least 30 minutes before serving to enable the flavors to mingle.

CHAPTER 2: LUNCH FOR SUSTAINING ENERGY

Quinoa Salad with Roasted Vegetables

Ingredients:

- For the Salad:
- 1 cup quinoa, rinsed and cooked according to package instructions
- 2 cups mixed vegetables, diced (such as bell peppers, zucchini, cherry tomatoes, and red onion)
- 2 tablespoons olive oil
- Salt and pepper to taste
- 1 teaspoon dried thyme (optional)
- For the Dressing:
- 3 tablespoons olive oil
- 2 tablespoons balsamic vinegar
- 1 teaspoon Dijon mustard

- 1 clove garlic, minced

- Salt and pepper to taste

- Additional Ingredients:

- 1/2 cup feta cheese, crumbled

- 1/4 cup fresh parsley, chopped

- 1/4 cup toasted pine nuts (optional)

Instructions:

1. Preheat the oven to 350°F.

2. Preheat the oven to 400 degrees Fahrenheit (200 degrees Celsius).

3. Vegetables to Roast: Toss the diced vegetables with olive oil, salt, pepper, and dried thyme (if using) in a large mixing dish.

   Arrange the vegetables in a single layer on a baking sheet.

   Roast for 20-25 minutes, or until the vegetables are soft and slightly caramelized, tossing halfway through.

4. Quinoa Cooking Instructions: Cold water should be used to rinse the quinoa, Cook the quinoa according to the package directions. Allow to cool after cooking.

5. Make the dressing: Whisk together olive oil, balsamic vinegar, Dijon mustard, minced garlic, salt, and pepper in a small bowl. Place aside.

6. Prepare the Salad: Combine the cooked quinoa and roasted vegetables in a large mixing basin.

7. Dress it up: Dress the quinoa and vegetables with the dressing. Gently toss everything to coat evenly.

8. Garnish: Sprinkle the salad with crumbled feta cheese, minced fresh parsley, and toasted pine nuts (if using).

9. Serve: At room temperature or cooled, serve the Quinoa Salad with Roasted Vegetables.

Chickpea and Spinach Stew

Ingredients:

- 2 tablespoons olive oil
- 1 large onion, finely chopped
- 3 cloves garlic, minced
- 1 teaspoon ground cumin
- 1 teaspoon ground coriander
- 1 teaspoon paprika
- 1/2 teaspoon ground turmeric
- 1/4 teaspoon cayenne pepper (adjust to taste)
- 1 can (15 oz) chickpeas, drained and rinsed
- 1 can (14 oz) diced tomatoes, undrained
- 1 cup vegetable broth
- 1 bay leaf
- Salt and pepper to taste
- 1 bunch fresh spinach, washed and chopped
- Juice of 1 lemon

- Fresh cilantro or parsley for garnish
- Cooked couscous or rice for serving

Instructions

1. Sauté the onions and garlic in the following order: Warm the olive oil in a big pot over medium heat. Sauté the chopped onions until they are transparent.

2. Spices to taste: Mix in the minced garlic, cumin, coriander, paprika, turmeric, and cayenne pepper. Cook for one minute, or until the spices become fragrant.

3. Toss in the chickpeas and tomatoes: To the pot, add chickpeas, diced tomatoes (with juices), vegetable broth, and bay leaf. Season to taste with salt and pepper.

4. Simmer: Bring the mixture to a boil, then lower to a low heat. enable it to simmer for 15-20 minutes to enable the flavors to mingle.

5. Spinach should be added: Cook until the spinach is wilted, stirring frequently. This should just take 3-5 minutes.

6. Finish with a squeeze of lemon juice: Squeeze one lemon's juice into the stew and mix well. If necessary, season with salt and pepper.

7. Serve: Remove and discard the bay leaf. Over cooked couscous or rice, serve the Chickpea and Spinach Stew.

8. Garnish: For a blast of freshness, garnish with fresh cilantro or parsley.

Stuffed Bell Peppers with Lentils and Brown Rice

Ingredients:

- 4 large bell peppers, halved and seeds removed
- 1 cup brown lentils, rinsed
- 1/2 cup brown rice, uncooked

- 2 1/2 cups vegetable broth
- 2 tablespoons olive oil
- 1 onion, finely chopped
- 2 cloves garlic, minced
- 1 carrot, diced
- 1 zucchini, diced
- 1 can (14 oz) diced tomatoes, drained
- 1 teaspoon ground cumin
- 1 teaspoon smoked paprika
- 1/2 teaspoon dried oregano
- Salt and pepper to taste
- 1 cup tomato sauce
- 1 cup shredded mozzarella or your favorite cheese
- Fresh parsley, chopped, for garnish

Instructions:

1. Preheat the oven to 350°F.
2. Preheat the oven to 375 degrees Fahrenheit (190 degrees Celsius).

3. Prepare the lentils and brown rice as follows: Brown lentils, brown rice, and vegetable broth should be combined in a medium-sized pot. Bring to a boil, then reduce to a low heat, cover, and cook until the lentils and rice are tender, about 25-30 minutes.

4. Vegetables Sauté: Warm the olive oil in a large skillet over medium heat. Chop the onion, mince the garlic, dice the carrot, and dice the zucchini. Cook for 5-7 minutes, or until the vegetables are softened.

5. Spices to taste: Add the ground cumin, smoked paprika, dried oregano, salt, and pepper to taste. Cook for another 2 minutes, or until the spices are fragrant.

6. Combine: In the skillet, combine the cooked lentils and brown rice. Mix in the drained diced tomatoes thoroughly.

7. Prepare the bell peppers as follows: In a baking dish, place the halved bell peppers. Fill each pepper half with the lentil and rice mixture.

8. Tomato sauce with cheese on top: Serve the stuffed peppers with tomato sauce. Top with shredded mozzarella or your chosen cheese.

9. Bake: Cover the baking dish tightly with aluminum foil and bake for 25-30 minutes, or until the peppers are cooked.

10. (Optional) Broil: Cover the dish and broil for a further 2-3 minutes, or until the cheese is lightly browned, if desired.

11. Garnish and serve with: Remove from the oven and top with freshly cut parsley. Serve the Stuffed Lentil and Brown Rice Bell Peppers warm.

Mushroom and Spinach Quiche

Ingredients:

- For the Pie Crust:
- 1 1/4 cups all-purpose flour
- 1/2 cup unsalted butter, cold and cubed
- 1/4 teaspoon salt
- 3-4 tablespoons ice water
-
- For the Filling:
- 1 tablespoon olive oil
- 1 small onion, finely chopped
- 2 cups mushrooms, sliced (button mushrooms or cremini)
- 2 cups fresh spinach, chopped
- 3 cloves garlic, minced
- Salt and pepper to taste
- 4 large eggs
- 1 cup milk (whole milk or half-and-half)
- 1 cup shredded Gruyere or Swiss cheese
- 1/2 cup grated Parmesan cheese

- 1/2 teaspoon dried thyme

- 1/4 teaspoon nutmeg (optional)

Instructions

1. For the pie crust, follow these steps:

2. Make the Pie Crust: Combine the flour, chilled butter cubes, and salt in a food processor. Pulse the ingredients until it resembles coarse crumbs.

3. One tablespoon at a time, add ice water and pulse until the dough comes together. Take care not to overmix.

4. Form the dough into a ball, flatten it into a disk, wrap it in plastic wrap, and place it in the refrigerator for at least 30 minutes.

5. Prepare the Crust: Preheat the oven to 375 degrees Fahrenheit (190 degrees Celsius).

6. Roll out the cold pie dough to fit a 9-inch pie plate on a floured surface. Transfer

the crust to the pie plate with care, pushing it into the bottom and up the edges.

7. Bake the Crust First: Fill the crust with pie weights or dry beans after lining it with parchment paper.

8. Bake for 12-15 minutes, or until the edges are just beginning to brown, in a preheated oven. Bake for an additional 5 minutes after removing the weights and parchment. Set aside after removing from the oven.

<u>To make the filling:</u>

9. Mushrooms with Spinach Sauté: Warm the olive oil in a pan over medium heat. Cook until the onions are softened. Cook until the mushrooms have released their moisture and turned golden brown. Mix in the spinach and garlic minced. Cook until the spinach begins to wilt. Season

with salt and pepper to taste. Allow the mixture to slightly cool.

10. Assemble the Quiche Filling: Whisk together the eggs, milk, shredded Gruyere or Swiss cheese, Parmesan cheese, dried thyme, and nutmeg (if using) in a mixing bowl. Stir in the mushroom and spinach combination that has been sautéed.

11. Prepare and bake: Fill the pie crust halfway with the quiche filling then Bake for 35-40 minutes, or until the centre is set and the top is golden brown, in a preheated oven.

12. Allow to cool before serving: Allow for a few minutes of cooling before slicing the Mushroom and Spinach Quiche.

Cauliflower and Chickpea Curry

Ingredients:

- 1 cauliflower, cut into florets
- 1 can (15 oz) chickpeas, drained and rinsed
- 1 large onion, finely chopped
- 3 cloves garlic, minced
- 1-inch piece of ginger, grated
- 2 tablespoons curry powder
- 1 teaspoon ground cumin
- 1 teaspoon ground coriander
- 1/2 teaspoon turmeric
- 1/4 teaspoon cayenne pepper (adjust to taste)
- 1 can (14 oz) diced tomatoes
- 1 can (14 oz) coconut milk
- 1 cup vegetable broth
- 1 tablespoon tomato paste
- 1 tablespoon olive oil
- Salt and pepper to taste
- Fresh cilantro, chopped (for garnish)
- Cooked basmati rice (for serving)

Introduction

1. Sauté the onions, garlic, and ginger as follows: Warm the olive oil in a big saucepan or deep skillet over medium heat. Cook until the onions are softened.

2. Sauté the minced garlic and grated ginger for an additional 1-2 minutes, or until fragrant.

3. Spices to taste: Stir in the curry powder, cumin, coriander, turmeric, and cayenne pepper. To toast the spices, cook for 1-2 minutes.

4. Cauliflower and chickpeas should be added: Fill the pot with cauliflower florets and drained chickpeas. Stir them thoroughly to coat them in the spice mixture.

5. Tomatoes, Coconut Milk, and Broth should be added at this point: Combine the diced tomatoes, coconut milk, and vegetable broth in a mixing bowl. Stir in

the tomato paste to mix. Season to taste
with salt and pepper.

6. Simmer: Bring the mixture to a boil, then
   lower to a low heat. Cover and cook for
   20-25 minutes, or until the cauliflower is
   soft.

7. Seasoning should be adjusted as follows:
   Season to taste, adding extra salt, pepper,
   or cayenne pepper as needed.

8. Serve: Over cooked basmati rice, serve
   the Cauliflower and Chickpea Curry.

9. Garnish: Before serving, garnish with
   chopped fresh cilantro.

Zucchini Noodles with Pesto and Cherry Tomatoes

Ingredients:

- For the Zucchini Noodles:
- 4 medium-sized zucchinis, spiralized into noodles

- 1 tablespoon olive oil

- Salt and pepper to taste

- For the Pesto:

- 2 cups fresh basil leaves, packed

- 1/2 cup grated Parmesan cheese

- 1/3 cup pine nuts or walnuts

- 2 cloves garlic, minced

- 1/2 cup extra-virgin olive oil

- Salt and pepper to taste

- For Assembly:

- 1 cup cherry tomatoes, halved

- Grated Parmesan cheese for topping

- Fresh basil leaves for garnish

Instructions

1. For the Zucchini Noodles, follow these steps:

2. Zucchini Spiralized: Spiralize the four medium-sized zucchinis to make zucchini noodles. If you don't have a

spiralizer, you can make ribbons with a vegetable peeler.

3. Prepare the Zucchini Noodles: In a large skillet over medium heat, heat 1 tablespoon olive oil. Sauté the zucchini noodles for 2-3 minutes, or until they are barely soft. Season to taste with salt and pepper.

4. Remove Excess Water: When cooked, zucchini noodles exude water. Drain and set aside any excess water from the pan.

5. To make the pesto:

6. Make the Pesto Sauce: Combine fresh basil, grated Parmesan cheese, pine nuts (or walnuts), and chopped garlic in a food processor.

7. Pulse the ingredients until finely minced.

8. Pour in the olive oil: Slowly pour in the extra-virgin olive oil while the food processor is running, until the pesto achieves the required consistency.

9. Season to taste with salt and pepper. Blend once more to combine.

10. For the Assembly:

11. Combine the Zucchini Noodles with the Pesto: Add the prepared pesto sauce to the pan with the cooked zucchini noodles. Toss the noodles until they are evenly covered.

12. Tomatoes, cherry: Gently mix in the halved cherry tomatoes and pesto to the zucchini noodles.

13. Serve: Serve the Zucchini Noodles with Pesto and Cherry Tomatoes on individual plates.

14. Garnish: To add color and taste, sprinkle with grated Parmesan cheese and fresh basil leaves.

Green Lentil Soup with Vegetables

Ingredients:

- 1 cup green lentils, rinsed and drained
- 1 large onion, finely chopped
- 2 carrots, peeled and diced
- 2 celery stalks, diced
- 3 cloves garlic, minced
- 1 can (14 oz) diced tomatoes
- 6 cups vegetable broth
- 1 teaspoon ground cumin
- 1 teaspoon ground coriander
- 1/2 teaspoon smoked paprika
- 1 bay leaf
- Salt and pepper to taste
- 2 tablespoons olive oil
- Juice of 1 lemon
- Fresh parsley, chopped (for garnish)
- Crusty bread (for serving)

Instructions

1. Aromatics: Sauté Instructions: Sauté: Warm the olive oil in a big pot over medium heat. Add the chopped onion, carrots, and celery. Cook for 5-7 minutes, or until the vegetables are softened.

2. Garlic and spices, if using: To the pot, add the minced garlic, ground cumin, ground coriander, smoked paprika, and bay leaf. Cook for a further 1-2 minutes, stirring frequently, until the spices are aromatic.

3. Pour in the lentils and broth: Add rinsed green lentils, diced tomatoes (with juices), and vegetable broth to the pot. To blend, stir everything together thoroughly.

4. Simmer: Bring the soup to a boil, then lower to a low heat. Cover the pot and cook for 25-30 minutes, or until the lentils are cooked.

5. Adjust and season: Season the soup to taste with salt and pepper. Season with salt and pepper to taste.

6. Finish with a squeeze of lemon juice: To brighten the tastes of the soup, add the juice of one lemon.

7. Serve: Pour the Green Lentil Soup with Vegetables into serving dishes.

8. Garnish: Garnish with fresh parsley, if desired.

9. Serve alongside Crusty Bread: For a complete and substantial lunch, serve the soup with crusty bread on the side.

CHAPTER 3: DINNERTIME

Quinoa Stuffed Bell Peppers

Ingredients:

- 4 large bell peppers, halved and seeds removed
- 1 cup quinoa, rinsed
- 2 cups vegetable broth
- 1 tablespoon olive oil
- 1 onion, finely chopped
- 2 cloves garlic, minced
- 1 zucchini, diced
- 1 carrot, grated
- 1 can (14 oz) diced tomatoes, drained
- 1 can (15 oz) black beans, drained and rinsed
- 1 teaspoon ground cumin
- 1 teaspoon smoked paprika
- Salt and pepper to taste

- 1 cup shredded cheese (cheddar, Monterey Jack, or a blend)
- Fresh cilantro or parsley for garnish

Instructions:

1. Preheat the oven to 350°F.
2. Preheat the oven to 375 degrees Fahrenheit (190 degrees Celsius).
3. Quinoa Cooking Instructions: Combine quinoa and vegetable broth in a medium saucepan. Bring to a boil, then lower to a low heat, cover, and leave to cook for 15-20 minutes, or until the quinoa is tender and the liquid has been absorbed.
4. Prepare the bell peppers as follows: Remove the seeds and membranes from the bell peppers by cutting them in half lengthwise. Put them in a baking pan.
5. Vegetables Sauté: Warm the olive oil in a large skillet over medium heat. Chop the onion, mince the garlic, cut the

zucchini, and grate the carrot. Cook the vegetables until they are tender.

6. Seasoning with Quinoa: Combine the cooked quinoa, drained diced tomatoes, black beans, ground cumin, smoked paprika, salt, and pepper in a mixing bowl. Cook for a further 2-3 minutes to allow the flavors to mingle.

7. Fill bell peppers with: Fill each bell pepper half with the quinoa mixture, carefully pressing down to pack the filling.

8. Serve with cheese: Shredded cheese should be sprinkled on top of each stuffed pepper.

9. Bake: Cover the baking dish tightly with aluminum foil and bake for 25-30 minutes, or until the peppers are cooked.

10. (Optional) Broil: Cover the dish and broil for a further 2-3 minutes, or until the cheese is lightly browned, if desired.

11. Garnish and serve with: Remove from the oven and sprinkle with fresh cilantro or parsley to serve.

Vegetable Stir-Fry with Tofu

Ingredients:

- For the Tofu:
- 1 block firm tofu, pressed and cubed
- 2 tablespoons soy sauce
- 1 tablespoon sesame oil
- 1 tablespoon cornstarch
- 1 tablespoon vegetable oil (for cooking tofu)
- For the Stir-Fry Sauce:
- 3 tablespoons soy sauce
- 2 tablespoons hoisin sauce
- 1 tablespoon rice vinegar
- 1 tablespoon sesame oil
- 1 tablespoon maple syrup or agave nectar

- 1 teaspoon cornstarch mixed with 2 teaspoons water (cornstarch slurry)
- For the Stir-Fry:
- 2 tablespoons vegetable oil
- 1 onion, thinly sliced
- 2 bell peppers, thinly sliced (use a mix of colors)
- 1 carrot, julienned
- 1 cup broccoli florets
- 1 cup snap peas, ends trimmed
- 3 cloves garlic, minced
- 1 tablespoon ginger, grated
- 4 cups cooked brown rice or quinoa (for serving)
- Sesame seeds and chopped green onions for garnish

Instructions:

1. To make the tofu:
2. Tofu Pressed and Cubed: Wrap the tofu in a clean kitchen towel and place a

heavy object on top for about 20-30 minutes to remove extra water. Cut the squeezed tofu into cubes.

3. Marinate the tofu: Combine the soy sauce, sesame oil, and cornstarch in a mixing dish. To coat, lightly toss in the cubed tofu. Allow at least 15-20 minutes for it to marinade.

4. Cooking Tofu: In a large skillet or wok, heat 1 tablespoon vegetable oil over medium-high heat. Cook until all sides of the marinated tofu are golden brown. Place aside.

5. Make the stir-fry sauce as follows: Stir-Fry Sauce: Whisk together soy sauce, hoisin sauce, rice vinegar, sesame oil, maple syrup (or agave nectar), and cornstarch slurry in a small basin. Place aside.

6. Make the Stir-Fry Vegetables:

7. Vegetables Sauté: Heat 2 tablespoons vegetable oil in the same skillet or wok over medium-high heat. Combine sliced onions, bell peppers, julienned carrots, broccoli florets, and snap peas in a mixing bowl. Stir-fry the vegetables for 3-5 minutes, or until they are slightly soft but still crisp.

8. Garlic and ginger, if using: Toss the vegetables with minced garlic and grated ginger. Stir-fry for another 1-2 minutes, or until aromatic.

9. Combine the tofu and the sauce: Put the cooked tofu back in the skillet. Serve the tofu and vegetables with the prepared stir-fry sauce. To coat evenly, toss everything together. Cook for another 2-3 minutes, or until the sauce thickens.

10. Serve: Serve the Tofu Vegetable Stir-Fry over cooked brown rice or quinoa.

11. Garnish: Garnish with sesame seeds and green onions, if desired.

Spinach and Chickpea Salad

Ingredients:

- For the Salad:
- 6 cups fresh baby spinach, washed and dried
- 1 can (15 oz) chickpeas, drained and rinsed
- 1 cup cherry tomatoes, halved
- 1 cucumber, diced
- 1/2 red onion, thinly sliced
- 1/2 cup feta cheese, crumbled (optional)
- 1/4 cup Kalamata olives, pitted and sliced (optional)
- For the Dressing:
- 3 tablespoons extra-virgin olive oil
- 2 tablespoons red wine vinegar

- 1 teaspoon Dijon mustard
- 1 clove garlic, minced
- 1 teaspoon honey or maple syrup
- Salt and pepper to taste
- Optional Additions:
- Grilled chicken or shrimp for added protein
- Avocado slices for creaminess

Introductions

1. Preparation of the Salad Base: Combine fresh baby spinach, drained and rinsed chickpeas, cherry tomatoes, diced cucumber, thinly sliced red onion, crumbled feta cheese, and sliced Kalamata olives in a large salad dish.

2. Prepare the Dressing: Whisk together extra-virgin olive oil, red wine vinegar, Dijon mustard, minced garlic, honey or maple syrup, salt, and pepper in a small

bowl. Season with salt and pepper to taste.

3. Prepare the Salad: Drizzle the salad dressing over the items.

4. Gently toss: Toss the salad carefully to coat all of the items evenly with the dressing.

5. Optional: Protein and creaminess can be added, Add grilled chicken or shrimp for extra protein if desired.
   You can also add slices of ripe avocado for smoothness.

6. Serve: Serve immediately with the Spinach and Chickpea Salad.

Lentil and Vegetable Soup

Ingredients:

- 1 cup dry brown lentils, rinsed

- 1 large onion, finely chopped
- 3 carrots, peeled and diced
- 3 celery stalks, diced
- 3 cloves garlic, minced
- 1 bell pepper, diced (any color)
- 1 zucchini, diced
- 1 can (14 oz) diced tomatoes, undrained
- 8 cups vegetable broth
- 2 teaspoons ground cumin
- 1 teaspoon ground coriander
- 1 teaspoon dried thyme
- 1 bay leaf
- Salt and pepper to taste
- 2 tablespoons olive oil
- Fresh parsley, chopped (for garnish)
- Lemon wedges (optional, for serving)

Instructions

1. Aromatics: Sauté Instructions: Sauté: Warm the olive oil in a big pot over medium heat. Add the chopped onion,

carrots, and celery. Cook for 5-7 minutes, or until the vegetables are softened.

2. Garlic and spices, if using: Mix in minced garlic, cumin, coriander, dry thyme, and a bay leaf. Cook for a further 1-2 minutes, stirring frequently, until the spices are aromatic.

3. Lentils and vegetables should be added: To the pot, add rinsed brown lentils, diced bell pepper, diced zucchini, and undrained diced tomatoes. To blend, stir everything together thoroughly.

4. Add the vegetable broth: Pour in the vegetable broth, making sure all of the ingredients are submerged. Season to taste with salt and pepper.

5. Simmer: Bring the soup to a boil, then lower to a low heat. Cover the pot and cook for 25-30 minutes, or until the lentils are cooked.

6. Seasoning should be adjusted as follows: Season to taste, adding more salt and pepper if necessary.

7. Serve: Pour the Lentil and Vegetable Soup into serving dishes.

8. Garnish: Garnish with fresh parsley, if desired.

9. Optional: Serve alongside Lemon Wedges:

10. Serve the soup with lemon wedges on the side for a blast of brightness.

Sweet Potato and Black Bean Chili

Ingredients:

- 2 medium sweet potatoes, peeled and diced

- 1 can (15 oz) black beans, drained and rinsed

- 1 large onion, diced

- 3 cloves garlic, minced

- 1 bell pepper, diced (any color)

- 1 jalapeño, seeded and minced (optional, for heat)

- 1 can (14 oz) diced tomatoes, undrained

- 1 can (14 oz) tomato sauce

- 2 cups vegetable broth

- 2 tablespoons chili powder

- 1 teaspoon ground cumin

- 1 teaspoon smoked paprika

- 1/2 teaspoon dried oregano

- 1/2 teaspoon ground coriander

- Salt and pepper to taste

- 2 tablespoons olive oil

- Fresh cilantro, chopped (for garnish)

- Avocado slices (for garnish, optional)

- Lime wedges (for serving)

Instructions

1. Aromatics: Sauté Instructions: Sauté: Warm the olive oil in a big pot over medium heat. Cook until the onion is softened, about 5 minutes.

2. Garlic and spices, if using: Mix in the garlic, chili powder, cumin, smoked paprika, dried oregano, and coriander. Cook for a further 1-2 minutes, stirring frequently, until the spices are aromatic.

3. Sweet potatoes and vegetables should be added: To the pot, add diced sweet potatoes, diced bell pepper, and minced jalapeo (if using). Toss the vegetables in the spice mixture to coat.

4. Add Tomatoes and Broth: Pour in the undrained diced tomatoes, tomato sauce, and vegetable broth. Bring the mixture to a low boil.

5. Simmer: Reduce the heat to low, cover, and leave to cook for 20-25 minutes, or until the sweet potatoes are cooked.

6. Add in the black beans: Mix in the rinsed and drained black beans. Cook for another 5-10 minutes, or until everything is well heated.

7. Adjust and season: Season the chili to taste with salt and pepper. If necessary, adjust the seasoning.

8. Serve: Fill bowls with the Sweet Potato and Black Bean Chili.

9. Garnish: If desired, garnish with chopped fresh cilantro and avocado slices.

10. Serve alongside Lime Wedges: Serve the chili with lime wedges on the side for a citrus kick.

Cauliflower Rice Bowl

Ingredients:

- For the Cauliflower Rice:

- 1 medium-sized cauliflower, grated or processed into rice-like texture
- 1 tablespoon olive oil
- Salt and pepper to taste
- 1 teaspoon garlic powder (optional)
- For the Bowl:
- Grilled or roasted vegetables of your choice (e.g., bell peppers, zucchini, cherry tomatoes)
- 1 cup cooked protein (e.g., grilled chicken, tofu, chickpeas)
- 1 avocado, sliced
- 1/4 cup hummus or tzatziki sauce (optional, for drizzling)
- Fresh herbs for garnish (e.g., cilantro, parsley, or chives)
- Sesame seeds or nuts for crunch (optional)

Instructions

1. For the Cauliflower Rice, follow these steps:

2. Cauliflower Rice Preparation: Use a box grater to grate the cauliflower, or process it in a food processor until it resembles rice.

3. Cauliflower Rice Sauté: Warm the olive oil in a large skillet over medium heat. If using, add the grated cauliflower, salt, pepper, and garlic powder. Sauté the cauliflower for 5-7 minutes, or until it is cooked but not mushy.

4. Keep aside: When the cauliflower rice is done, set it aside.

5. Putting Together the Bowl:

6. Vegetables, grilled or roasted: Grill or roast your preferred vegetables until soft and faintly browned. Season with salt and pepper to taste.

7. Protein Preparation: Cook your preferred protein (grilled chicken, tofu, or

chickpeas) according to package directions.

8. Prepare the Bowl: Arrange cauliflower rice, grilled or roasted veggies, and your preferred protein in serving bowls.

9. Include Avocado: To add creaminess, top the bowl with sliced avocado.

10. Drizzle with the following sauce: To add flavor, drizzle hummus or tzatziki sauce over the bowl.

11. Garnish: For a burst of freshness and crunch, garnish with fresh herbs, sesame seeds, or nuts.

Mushroom and Spinach Stuffed Portobello Mushrooms

Ingredients:

- 4 large Portobello mushrooms, stems removed and cleaned
- 2 tablespoons olive oil
- 1 onion, finely chopped
- 2 cloves garlic, minced
- 2 cups baby spinach, chopped
- 2 cups mushrooms, finely chopped (use a variety such as cremini or button mushrooms)
- 1/2 cup breadcrumbs
- 1/2 cup grated Parmesan cheese
- 1/4 cup fresh parsley, chopped
- Salt and pepper to taste
- 1 cup shredded mozzarella cheese (optional, for topping)
- Fresh thyme or additional parsley for garnish

Instructions

1. Preheat the oven to 350°F.

2. Preheat the oven to 375 degrees Fahrenheit (190 degrees Celsius).

3. Prepare the Portobello Mushrooms as follows: Remove the stems from the Portobello mushrooms. Place them, gill side up, on a baking sheet.

4. Onion and garlic sauté: Warm the olive oil in a pan over medium heat. Sauté the finely chopped onion until softened. Cook for an additional 1-2 minutes, or until the garlic is aromatic.

5. Mushrooms and spinach, optional: Cook until the mushrooms release their moisture and become soft, about 5 minutes. Cook until the baby spinach has wilted. Season to taste with salt and pepper.

6. Make the filling: Combine the sautéed mushroom and spinach mixture with the breadcrumbs, grated Parmesan cheese, and chopped fresh parsley in a mixing

dish. To make a stuffing, thoroughly combine all of the ingredients.

7. Portobello Mushroom Stuffing: Fill each Portobello mushroom cap with the prepared stuffing and gently push it down.

8. Optional: Mozzarella on top: For a delicious touch, add shredded mozzarella cheese on top of each stuffed mushroom.

9. Bake: Bake for 20-25 minutes, or until the mushrooms are soft and the filling is golden brown, in a preheated oven.

10. Garnish and serve with: Remove from the oven and top with fresh thyme or more parsley.

11. Serve hot: Warm Portobello Mushrooms with Mushroom and Spinach Stuffing.

Zucchini Noodles with Pesto

Ingredients:

- For the Zucchini Noodles:
- 4 medium-sized zucchinis, spiralized into noodles
- 1 tablespoon olive oil
- Salt and pepper to taste
- For the Pesto:
- 2 cups fresh basil leaves, packed
- 1/2 cup grated Parmesan cheese
- 1/3 cup pine nuts or walnuts
- 2 cloves garlic, minced
- 1/2 cup extra-virgin olive oil
- Salt and pepper to taste
- Juice of 1 lemon (optional, for added freshness)

Instructions

1. To make the Zucchini Noodles:

2. Zucchini Spiralized: Spiralize the four medium-sized zucchinis to make zucchini noodles. If you don't have a spiralizer, you can make ribbons with a vegetable peeler.

3. Prepare the Zucchini Noodles: 1 tablespoon olive oil, heated in a large skillet over medium heat. Sauté the zucchini noodles for 2-3 minutes, or until they are barely soft. Season to taste with salt and pepper.

4. Remove Excess Water: When cooked, zucchini noodles exude water. Set aside any surplus water from the skillet.

5. To make the pesto:

6. Make the Pesto Sauce: Combine fresh basil, grated Parmesan cheese, pine nuts (or walnuts), chopped garlic, and a touch of salt and pepper in a food processor.

7. Blend: While the food processor is running, carefully drizzle in the extra-

virgin olive oil until the pesto is the consistency you want. If necessary, add more olive oil.

8. Seasoning should be adjusted as follows: Taste the pesto and season with salt and pepper to taste. Add the juice of one lemon and blend again if you prefer a bit of acidity.

9. Prepare the Dish:

10. Toss together pesto and zucchini noodles: Add the prepared pesto sauce to the skillet with the cooked zucchini noodles. Toss the noodles in the pesto until evenly coated.

11. Serve: Serve the Zucchini Noodles with Pesto on plates.

12. Optional garnish: Garnish with more grated Parmesan cheese and fresh basil leaves, if desired.

Black Bean and Vegetable Soup

Ingredients:

- 1 can (15 oz) black beans, drained and rinsed
- 1 tablespoon olive oil
- 1 onion, finely chopped
- 3 cloves garlic, minced
- 1 carrot, diced
- 1 bell pepper (any color), diced
- 1 zucchini, diced
- 1 cup corn kernels (fresh, frozen, or canned)
- 1 can (14 oz) diced tomatoes
- 4 cups vegetable broth
- 1 teaspoon ground cumin
- 1 teaspoon chili powder
- 1/2 teaspoon smoked paprika
- Salt and pepper to taste
- 1 lime, juiced
- Fresh cilantro, chopped (for garnish)

- Avocado slices (for serving)
- Sour cream or Greek yogurt (optional, for serving)

Instructions

1. Aromatics for Sauté: Warm the olive oil in a big pot over medium heat. Sauté the chopped onion until softened. Cook for an additional 1-2 minutes, or until the garlic is aromatic.

2. Include Vegetables: To the pot, add diced carrot, diced bell pepper, diced zucchini, and corn kernels. Cook for 5 minutes, or until the vegetables soften.

3. Season: Add the ground cumin, chili powder, smoked paprika, salt, and pepper to taste. Mix thoroughly to coat the vegetables in the seasonings.

4. Toss in the black beans and tomatoes: To the pot, add drained and rinsed black beans, chopped tomatoes (with juices),

and vegetable broth. To blend, stir everything together.

5. Simmer: Bring the soup to a boil, then lower to a low heat. Allow the flavors to mingle by covering the pot and simmering for 20-25 minutes.

6. Seasoning should be adjusted as follows: Season with salt and pepper to taste. If you like your soup with a little acidity, squeeze the juice of one lime into it and stir it in.

7. Serve: Pour the Black Bean and Vegetable Soup into serving dishes.

8. Garnish: Garnish with fresh cilantro, if desired.

9. Optional: Toppings are optional: If preferred, top each dish with avocado slices and a dollop of sour cream or Greek yogurt.

CHAPTER 4: SNACKS AND APPETIZERS

Roasted Chickpeas

Ingredients:

- 2 cans (15 oz each) chickpeas, drained and rinsed (or 3 cups cooked chickpeas)
- 2 tablespoons olive oil
- 1 teaspoon ground cumin
- 1 teaspoon smoked paprika
- 1/2 teaspoon garlic powder
- 1/2 teaspoon onion powder
- 1/4 teaspoon cayenne pepper (adjust to taste for spiciness)
- Salt and pepper to taste

Instructions:

1. Preheat the oven to 350°F.

2. Preheat the oven to 400 degrees Fahrenheit (200 degrees Celsius).

3. Chickpeas, dried: Drain and thoroughly rinse the chickpeas. To eliminate any excess moisture, pat them dry with a paper towel.

4. Chickpeas should be seasoned as follows: Toss the chickpeas with olive oil, ground cumin, smoked paprika, garlic powder, onion powder, cayenne pepper, salt, and pepper in a large mixing bowl. Make sure the chickpeas are well coated with the seasonings.

5. Spread out on a baking sheet: On a baking sheet lined with parchment paper, spread the seasoned chickpeas in a single layer. This helps to reduce stickiness and makes cleanup easier.

6. Bake in the Oven: Roast the chickpeas for 25-30 minutes in a preheated oven, stirring the pan halfway through to

ensure even roasting. Chickpeas should turn golden brown and crunchy.

7. Allow to cool before serving: Allow the roasted chickpeas to cool slightly before serving. As they cool, they will continue to crisp up.

8. Optional Substitutions: Experiment with other seasonings such as curry powder, turmeric, cajun seasoning, or your favorite herbs and spices.

9. Store: Leftover roasted chickpeas can be stored in an airtight jar at room temperature for up to a week. You can reheat them in the oven for a few minutes if they lose their crispiness.

Vegetable Crudites with Hummus

Ingredients:

- For the Hummus:

- 1 can (15 oz) chickpeas, drained and rinsed
- 1/4 cup tahini
- 2 tablespoons lemon juice
- 2 cloves garlic, minced
- 1/2 teaspoon ground cumin
- 1/4 teaspoon smoked paprika
- Salt and pepper to taste
- 1/4 cup extra-virgin olive oil
- Water (as needed to adjust consistency)
- For the Vegetable Crudites:
- Carrot sticks
- Cucumber slices
- Bell pepper strips (assorted colors)
- Cherry tomatoes
- Celery sticks
- Broccoli florets
- Radishes, sliced
- Any other favorite raw vegetables

Instructions

1. To make the Hummus:

2. Prepare the chickpeas as follows:Drain and thoroughly rinse the chickpeas.

3. Blend Ingredients: Combine chickpeas, tahini, lemon juice, minced garlic, ground cumin, smoked paprika, salt, and pepper in a food processor.

4. Blend until completely smooth: Blend the ingredients together until smooth. While the food processor is running, sprinkle in the olive oil slowly. If the hummus is too thick, add a tablespoon of water at a time until it reaches the appropriate consistency.

5. Seasoning should be adjusted as follows: Seasoning should be tasted and adjusted to taste. If necessary, add extra lemon juice, salt, or pepper.

6. Keep aside: Put the hummus in a serving bowl and set it aside.

7. For the Crudites de légumes:

8. Vegetable Preparation: Wash the vegetables and cut them into sticks, slices, or bite-sized pieces.

9. Arrange the following on a platter: Arrange the veggie crudites on a dish to serve.

10. Serve alongside Hummus: Place the hummus bowl in the center of the platter or on one side.

11. Optional garnish: Garnish the hummus with olive oil, smoked paprika, or a few chopped fresh herbs such as parsley or cilantro.

12. Serve: As a nutritious and savory appetizer or snack, serve the Vegetable Crudites with Hummus.

Stuffed Grape Leaves

Ingredients:

- For the Filling:

- 1 cup short-grain rice, washed and drained
- 1/2 cup pine nuts
- 1/2 cup currants or chopped raisins
- 1 medium onion, finely chopped
- 2 tablespoons olive oil
- 1/2 cup fresh parsley, finely chopped
- 1/4 cup fresh dill, finely chopped
- Salt and pepper to taste
- For the Grape Leaves:
- 1 jar preserved grape leaves in brine, drained and rinsed
- Juice of 2 lemons
- For Cooking:
- 2 cups vegetable broth or water
- 1/4 cup olive oil

Instructions

1. Getting the Grape Leaves Ready:
2. Grape Leaves Soak: Fill a large basin halfway with boiling water and add the

grape leaves. Allow them to soak for 10-15 minutes to soften. Drain and rinse them under cold water.

3. Trim the stems: Remove the grape leaves' stiff stalks.

4. Make the Filling: Combine the washed and drained rice, pine nuts, currants or raisins, finely chopped onion, olive oil, chopped parsley, chopped dill, salt, and pepper in a large mixing dish. Combine thoroughly.

5. Gather the Dolma: Place a grape leaf flat on a clean surface, glossy side down, stem side facing you. Place a tablespoon of the filling toward the leaf's stem end.

6. Dolma, roll the dice: Fold the bottom of the leaf over the filling, then the sides, and tightly roll into a cigar-shaped packet.

7. Repeat: Repeat with the rest of the grape leaves and filling.

8. Preparing the Dolma:

9. Layer in the pot: Make a layer of any damaged or unused grape leaves at the bottom of a large pot. This aids in the prevention of sticking.

10. Arrange for Dolma: Layer the rolled grape leaves in the pot, seam side down. Put them together securely to prevent them from unraveling while cooking.

11. Pour in the liquid: Combine the vegetable broth or water, olive oil, and lemon juice in a mixing bowl. This mixture should be poured over the packed grape leaves.

12. Simmer: Cover and cook over low heat for 45-50 minutes, or until the rice is done and the grape leaves are soft.

13. Allow to cool before serving: Allow to cool before presenting the packed grape leaves. They can be served either warm or cold.

Cauliflower Wings

Ingredients:

- For the Cauliflower:
- 1 large head of cauliflower, cut into florets
- 1 cup all-purpose flour
- 1 cup plant-based milk (such as almond, soy, or oat milk)
- 1 teaspoon garlic powder
- 1 teaspoon onion powder
- 1/2 teaspoon smoked paprika
- 1/2 teaspoon salt
- 1/4 teaspoon black pepper
- For the Buffalo Sauce:
- 1/2 cup hot sauce (such as Frank's RedHot)
- 1/4 cup melted vegan butter
- 1 tablespoon maple syrup or agave nectar
- 1 teaspoon garlic powder
- 1 teaspoon onion powder

- Optional for Serving:
- Celery sticks
- Carrot sticks
- Vegan ranch or blue cheese dressing

Instructions

1. Cauliflower preparation:
2. Preheat the oven to 350°F.
3. Preheat the oven to 450 degrees Fahrenheit (230 degrees Celsius).
4. Make the batter: In a large mixing bowl, combine the flour, plant-based milk, garlic powder, onion powder, smoked paprika, salt, and black pepper until smooth.
5. Cauliflower Coat: Dip each cauliflower floret into the batter, coating well. Allow any remaining batter to trickle off.
6. Bake: Line a baking sheet with parchment paper and place the battered cauliflower on it. Bake for 20-25

minutes, or until the cauliflower is golden and crisp, in a preheated oven.

7. To make the Buffalo Sauce:

8. Sauce Combination: Combine spicy sauce, melted vegan butter, maple syrup or agave nectar, garlic powder, and onion powder in a separate bowl.

9. Cauliflower Coat: When the cauliflower is done baking, place it in a large mixing dish. Pour the buffalo sauce over the cauliflower and toss until evenly coated.

10. Bake once more: Return the sauced cauliflower to the baking sheet and bake for another 10-15 minutes, or until the cauliflower is crispy and the sauce has caramelized.

11. Optional: Broil (for additional crispiness): Broil for 1-2 minutes for added crispiness, looking carefully to avoid scorching.

12. Serve:

13. Slightly cool: Allow the Cauliflower Wings to cool for a few minutes before serving.

14. Serve with the following dipping sauce: Serve the Cauliflower Wings with celery and carrot sticks for dipping, as well as your favorite vegan ranch or blue cheese dressing.

Sweet Potato Bites

Ingredients:

- For the Sweet Potato Bites:
- 2 medium-sized sweet potatoes, peeled and sliced into rounds
- 2 tablespoons olive oil
- 1 teaspoon smoked paprika
- 1/2 teaspoon garlic powder
- 1/2 teaspoon onion powder
- Salt and pepper to taste
- For the Topping:

- 1/2 cup black beans, drained and rinsed

- 1/2 cup corn kernels (fresh, frozen, or canned)

- 1/4 cup red onion, finely chopped

- 1/4 cup fresh cilantro, chopped

- Juice of 1 lime

- Salt and pepper to taste

- Optional Garnish:

- Avocado slices

- Vegan sour cream or yogurt

Instructions

1. For the Sweet Potato Bites, prepare the following:

2. Preheat the oven to 350°F.

3. Preheat the oven to 400 degrees Fahrenheit (200 degrees Celsius).

4. Sweet potatoes should be prepared as follows: Peel the sweet potatoes and cut them into 1/4-inch thick rounds.

5. Sweet potatoes should be seasoned as follows: Toss the sweet potato rounds with olive oil, smoked paprika, garlic powder, onion powder, salt, and pepper in a large mixing bowl. Make sure the sweet potato rounds are covered evenly.

6. Bake: Line a baking sheet with parchment paper and place the seasoned sweet potato rounds on it. Bake for 20-25 minutes, or until the sweet potatoes are soft and slightly crispy around the edges.

7. For the icing:

8. Make the toppings: In a mixing bowl, combine black beans, corn, red onion, cilantro, and lime juice. Season to taste with salt and pepper.

9. Assemble: When the sweet potato rounds are done, put a spoonful of the black bean and corn mixture on top of each one.

10. Optional: Garnish: If preferred, garnish with avocado slices and a dollop of vegan sour cream or yogurt.

11. Serve: Serve the Sweet Potato Bites immediately on a serving plate.

Edamame Guacamole

Ingredients:

- 1 cup shelled edamame, cooked and cooled
- 2 ripe avocados, peeled and pitted
- 1/4 cup red onion, finely chopped
- 1/4 cup fresh cilantro, chopped
- 1 jalapeño, seeds removed and finely chopped (optional, for heat)
- 2 cloves garlic, minced
- Juice of 1 lime
- Salt and pepper to taste
- 1/2 teaspoon ground cumin (optional)

- Tortilla chips or vegetable sticks for serving

Instructions

1. Make Edamame: Shelled edamame should be cooked according per package directions. After cooking, drain and cool.

2. Avocado Mash: Mash the ripe avocados with a fork or potato masher in a medium-sized mixing bowl until they are smooth.

3. Combine the following ingredients: To the mashed avocados, add the cooled edamame, chopped red onion, cilantro, jalapeo (if using), minced garlic, and lime juice.

4. Season: Season the guacamole with salt, pepper, and (if using) ground cumin. Adjust the seasoning to suit your taste.

5. Combine thoroughly: Mix all of the ingredients together until they are uniformly distributed.

6. Garnish, if desired: For a decorative touch, top the Edamame Guacamole with more cilantro and a few whole edamame beans.

7. Optional chilling: If you have time, cover and chill the guacamole for 30 minutes to enable the flavors to mingle.

8. Serve: With tortilla chips or veggie sticks, serve the Edamame Guacamole.

Mushroom and Spinach Phyllo Cups

Ingredients:

- 1 package (15 sheets) phyllo dough, thawed if frozen
- 2 tablespoons olive oil
- 1 onion, finely chopped

- 2 cloves garlic, minced

- 8 oz (about 225g) mushrooms, finely chopped

- 4 cups fresh spinach, chopped

- Salt and pepper to taste

- 1/2 cup feta cheese, crumbled (optional)

- 1/4 cup grated Parmesan cheese

- 1/3 cup ricotta cheese

- 1/4 teaspoon nutmeg (optional, for extra flavor)

- Cooking spray or additional olive oil for brushing phyllo dough

Instructions:

1. Preheat the oven:

2. Preheat the oven to 375 degrees Fahrenheit (190 degrees Celsius).

3. Make the Phyllo Cups: Spread the phyllo dough sheets out on a clean board. Cover them with a damp kitchen towel to keep them from drying out while you work.

Cut the sheets to fit if they are larger than your muffin tin cups.

4. Filling with Sautéed Mushrooms and Spinach: Warm the olive oil in a pan over medium heat. Cook until the onion has softened. Mix in the minced garlic and chopped mushrooms. Cook the mushrooms until they release their liquid and become soft. Cook until the spinach is wilted, about 5 minutes. Season with salt and pepper to taste.

5. Remove Excess Liquid: Drain any excess liquid from the mushroom and spinach mixture to avoid making the phyllo cups soggy.

6. Make the Cheese Mixture: Combine crumbled feta (if using), grated Parmesan, ricotta cheese, and nutmeg in a mixing bowl. Combine thoroughly.

7. Fillings should be combined: To the cheese mixture, add the sautéed

mushroom and spinach mixture. Mix until all of the ingredients are thoroughly incorporated.

8. Make the Phyllo Cups: Coat each muffin cup lightly with cooking spray or brush with olive oil. In each cup, layer three sheets of phyllo dough, rotating them slightly to ensure even coverage.

9. Fill Phyllo cups as follows: Distribute the mushroom and spinach filling evenly among the phyllo cups.

10. Folding and sealing: Fold and scrunch the phyllo dough gently over the filling to form a cup-like shape. Seal the edges to prevent them from unraveling during baking.

11. Bake: Bake for 15-20 minutes, or until the phyllo cups are golden brown and crispy, in a preheated oven.

12. Slightly cool: Before serving, let the Mushroom and Spinach Phyllo Cups to cool slightly.

13. Serve: As an appetizer or side dish, serve warm.

Cucumber Avocado Rolls

Ingredients:

- 2 large cucumbers
- 1 ripe avocado
- 1/2 cup cherry tomatoes, diced
- 1/4 cup red onion, finely chopped
- 1/4 cup fresh cilantro, chopped
- Juice of 1 lime
- Salt and pepper to taste
- Sesame seeds for garnish (optional)
- Soy sauce or tamari for dipping

Instructions

1. Cucumbers should be prepared as follows: Thoroughly wash the cucumbers. Slice the cucumbers lengthwise into thin, long strips using a vegetable peeler. A mandoline slicer can also be used for precision.

2. Make the Avocado Filling: Mash the ripe avocado in a bowl. Diced cherry tomatoes, finely chopped red onion, cilantro, lime juice, salt, and pepper to taste. Mix the ingredients together to make a guacamole-like filling.

3. Assemble the Rolls: Spread a cucumber strip on a clean surface. Fill one end of the cucumber strip with a small bit of the avocado filling.

4. Roll it up: Roll the cucumber strip carefully around the avocado filling to form a tiny roll or sushi-like shape. Repeat with the rest of the cucumber strips and filling.

5. Optional: Garnish: To add texture and taste, sprinkle sesame seeds on top of the cucumber avocado rolls.

6. Optional chilling: Chill the cucumber avocado rolls in the refrigerator for 15-20 minutes before serving for a refreshing touch.

7. Cut and serve: Cut the rolls into bite-sized pieces with a sharp knife. Place them on a serving platter.

8. Serve with the following dipping sauce: Serve the Cucumber Avocado Rolls with a dipping sauce of soy sauce or tamari.

Spicy Roasted Nuts

Ingredients:

- 2 cups mixed nuts (such as almonds, cashews, walnuts, and pecans)
- 1 tablespoon olive oil

- 1 tablespoon maple syrup or honey

- 1 teaspoon ground cumin

- 1 teaspoon paprika

- 1/2 teaspoon cayenne pepper (adjust to taste for spiciness)

- 1/2 teaspoon garlic powder

- 1/2 teaspoon onion powder

- 1 teaspoon sea salt (adjust to taste)

- Freshly ground black pepper to taste

Instructions:

1. Preheat the oven to 350°F.

2. Preheat the oven to 350 degrees Fahrenheit (175 degrees Celsius).

3. Make the Nuts: Combine the mixed nuts, olive oil, and maple syrup or honey in a large mixing basin. Toss to evenly coat the nuts.

4. Spices to taste: Combine ground cumin, paprika, cayenne pepper, garlic powder,

onion powder, sea salt, and black pepper
in a small bowl.

5. Nuts for Coats: To ensure that all of the
   nuts are coated with the spicy seasoning,
   sprinkle the spice mixture over them and
   toss well.

6. Bake in the Oven: On a baking sheet
   lined with parchment paper, spread the
   seasoned nuts in a single layer.

7. Roast: Roast for 12-15 minutes in a
   warm oven, stirring halfway through to
   ensure equal roasting. To avoid burning,
   keep a tight eye on them.

8. Cool: Allow the Spicy Roasted Nuts on
   the baking sheet to cool fully. As they
   cool, they will continue to crisp up.

9. Store: Transfer the nuts to an airtight
   container once they have totally cooled.
   They can be kept at room temperature
   for two weeks.

10. Serve and have fun: As a tasty snack or appetizer, serve these Spicy Roasted Nuts. They're also delicious on cheese boards or as a salad topping.

11. Adjust the level of heat: Feel free to modify the spice amounts to your personal taste. Increase the cayenne pepper for greater heat, or decrease it for a softer flavor.

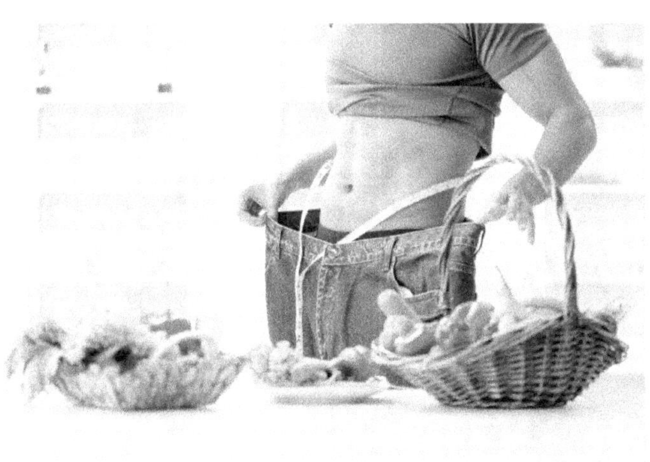

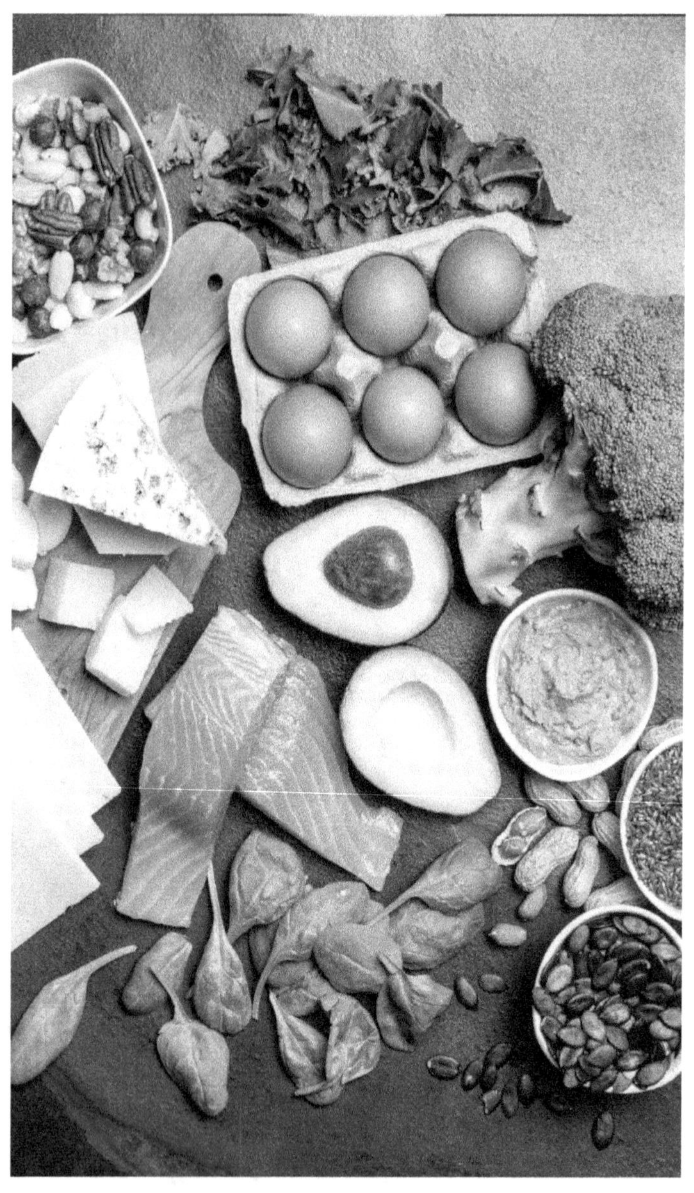

CHAPTER 5: SWEET TREATS WITHOUT GUIT

Chocolate Avocado Mousse

Ingredients:

- 2 ripe avocados, peeled and pitted
- 1/2 cup unsweetened cocoa powder
- 1/2 cup maple syrup or agave nectar
- 1/3 cup coconut milk (or any plant-based milk)
- 1 teaspoon vanilla extract
- A pinch of salt
- Optional toppings: Fresh berries, chopped nuts, or coconut flakes

Instructions:

1. Avocados should be prepared as follows: Place the flesh from the ripe avocados in a blender or food processor.

2. Mix with the cocoa powder: To the blender, add the unsweetened cocoa powder.

3. Use maple syrup to sweeten: Pour in the maple syrup or agave nectar to make it sweeter.

4. Add the Coconut Milk: Pour in the coconut milk (or your preferred plant-based milk).

5. Pour in the vanilla extract: Add the vanilla extract and a bit of salt to taste.

6. Blend until completely smooth: Blend all of the ingredients until they are smooth and creamy. As needed, scrape down the sides of the blender or food processor.

7. Adjust to taste: If necessary, alter the sweetness or cocoa intensity of the chocolate avocado mixture. You can adjust the sweetness and cocoa powder to your liking.

8. Optional chilling: Refrigerate the mixture for at least 30 minutes before serving for a richer mousse and to enhance the taste.

9. Serve: Fill serving plates or glasses halfway with the Chocolate Avocado Mousse.

10. Optional garnish: For extra texture and flavor, garnish with fresh berries, chopped nuts, or coconut flakes.

Berry Nice Cream

Ingredients:

- 3 ripe bananas, sliced and frozen
- 1 cup mixed berries (such as strawberries, blueberries, and raspberries), frozen

- 1-2 tablespoons maple syrup or agave nectar (optional, for added sweetness)
- 1 teaspoon vanilla extract (optional)
- Fresh berries, mint leaves, or granola for garnish (optional)

Instructions:

1. Bananas and berries can be frozen:
2. Put ripe bananas on a plate or in a container lined with parchment paper. Mix in the berries. Freeze for at least four hours, preferably overnight.
3. Frozen Fruit Blend: Add the frozen banana slices and mixed berries to a high-powered blender or food processor. Allow the fruits to soften for a few minutes at room temperature if necessary.
4. Blend until completely smooth: Blend until the frozen fruits are smooth and creamy. You may need to pause the

blender or food processor a few times to scrape down the sides.

5. (Optional):

6. sweeten: If you want more sweetness, add maple syrup or agave nectar to the excellent cream. If desired, add vanilla extract for added taste. Blend once more to integrate.

7. Serve right away: Fill bowls or cones with Berry Nice Cream.

8. Optional garnish: For extra texture and presentation, garnish with fresh berries, mint leaves, or granola.

Date and Nut Energy Bites

Ingredients:

- 1 cup pitted dates

- 1 cup mixed nuts (such as almonds, walnuts, or cashews)
- 1/4 cup shredded coconut (unsweetened)
- 1 tablespoon chia seeds
- 1 tablespoon flaxseeds
- 1 teaspoon vanilla extract
- A pinch of salt (optional)
- Additional shredded coconut or finely chopped nuts for coating (optional)

Instructions

1. Dates for preparation: Soak the dates in warm water for about 10 minutes if they are not soft. Drain thoroughly.
2. Combine the following ingredients: Combine dates, mixed nuts, shredded coconut, chia seeds, flaxseeds, vanilla essence, and a pinch of salt (if using) in a food processor.
3. Continue to process until a sticky dough forms: Mix the ingredients together until

a sticky dough forms. Finely chop the nuts, and the mixture should hold together easily when pushed between your fingers.

4. Bite Forms: Roll little amounts of the mixture between your palms to form bite-sized balls. If the mixture is excessively sticky, softly wet your hands.

5. Coating Options: Roll the energy bites in extra shredded coconut or finely chopped nuts to cover the outside if desired.

6. Optional chilling: Refrigerate the energy bites for at least 30 minutes before serving for firmer bites.

7. Store: Refrigerate the Date and Nut Energy Bites in an airtight container for up to two weeks. You can even freeze them for longer periods of time.

Coconut Chia Pudding

Ingredients:

- 1/4 cup chia seeds
- 1 cup coconut milk (canned, full-fat for creaminess)
- 1 tablespoon maple syrup or sweetener of choice
- 1/2 teaspoon vanilla extract
- Shredded coconut and fresh berries for topping (optional)

Instructions:

1. Chia Seeds and Coconut Milk should be combined: Combine the chia seeds, coconut milk, maple syrup, and vanilla extract in a mixing dish.
2. Thoroughly whisk: To ensure that the chia seeds are evenly dispersed and do not clump together, carefully whisk the mixture.

3. Refrigerate: Refrigerate the mixture for at least 4 hours, preferably overnight. The chia seeds will absorb the liquid and form a pudding-like consistency during this time.

4. (Optional) Stir: Stir the mixture again after about 30 minutes in the refrigerator to prevent clumping.

5. Examine Consistency: Check the consistency before serving. If the pudding is too thick, mix in a little more coconut milk until thoroughly incorporated.

6. Serve: Fill serving cups or jars halfway with the Coconut Chia Pudding.

7. Top with optional toppings: To enhance flavor and texture, top with shredded coconut and fresh berries.

Baked Cinnamon Apples

Ingredients:

- 4 large apples (such as Honeycrisp or Granny Smith), cored and sliced
- 2 tablespoons unsalted butter, melted (or coconut oil for a dairy-free option)
- 2 tablespoons maple syrup or honey
- 1 teaspoon ground cinnamon
- 1/4 teaspoon ground nutmeg
- 1/4 teaspoon vanilla extract
- A pinch of salt
- Optional toppings: Chopped nuts, raisins, or a dollop of yogurt

Instructions:

1. Preheat the oven to 350°F.
2. Preheat the oven to 375 degrees Fahrenheit (190 degrees Celsius).
3. Prepare the apples: Apples should be peeled and sliced into thin wedges. Keep

the peel on for additional texture and nutrition.

4. Combine the following ingredients: Melted butter, maple syrup or honey, ground cinnamon, ground nutmeg, vanilla essence, and a pinch of salt should be combined in a large mixing basin.

5. Apple Coat: Combine the cut apples with the cinnamon mixture in a mixing dish. Toss until the apples are thoroughly covered.

6. Place in a baking dish: Place the coated apples in a baking dish and spread them out evenly.

7. Bake: Bake for 25-30 minutes, or until the apples are soft and slightly caramelized, stirring halfway through, in a preheated oven.

8. Optional Extras: Sprinkle chopped nuts or raisins over the baked apples during the last 5 minutes of baking if desired.

9. Slightly cool: Allow the Baked Cinnamon Apples to cool for a few minutes before serving.

10. Serve: Fill serving bowls halfway with cooked apples. To add a wonderful contrast, top with a dollop of yogurt.

Pumpkin Spice Smoothie

Ingredients:

- 1/2 cup canned pumpkin puree
- 1 ripe banana, frozen
- 1/2 cup plain Greek yogurt (or non-dairy yogurt for a vegan option)
- 1/2 cup almond milk (or any milk of your choice)

- 1 tablespoon maple syrup or honey (adjust to taste)
- 1/2 teaspoon pumpkin pie spice
- 1/2 teaspoon vanilla extract
- 1/2 cup ice cubes
- Optional toppings: Whipped cream, a sprinkle of cinnamon, or crushed graham crackers

Instructions:

1. Combine the following ingredients: Blend the canned pumpkin puree, frozen banana, Greek yogurt, almond milk, maple syrup or honey, pumpkin pie spice, and vanilla extract in a blender until smooth.

2. Blend until completely smooth: Blend until the mixture is smooth and creamy. If the smoothie is too thick, add more almond milk in small amounts until the ideal consistency is reached.

3. Adjust to taste: Taste the smoothie and adjust the sweetness as needed by adding more maple syrup or honey.

4. Add the ice cubes: Blend in the ice cubes again until the smoothie is thoroughly cold.

5. Serve: Fill glasses halfway with Pumpkin Spice Smoothie.

6. Optional Extras: For a festive touch, top the smoothie with a dollop of whipped cream, a sprinkling of cinnamon, or crushed graham crackers.

Almond Butter Banana Bites

Ingredients:

- 2 ripe bananas
- 1/4 cup almond butter (or any nut or seed butter of your choice)

- 1/4 cup granola

- 2 tablespoons shredded coconut

- 1-2 tablespoons dark chocolate chips (optional)

- Chopped nuts (such as almonds or walnuts) for garnish (optional)

Instructions

1. Prepare the bananas as follows: Peel the bananas and cut them into 1/2-inch thick bite-sized rounds.

2. Make the Banana Bites: Top each banana round with a thin coating of almond butter.

3. Granola on top: Sprinkle granola on top of each banana round and gently push it into the almond butter to adhere.

4. Toss in the shredded coconut: On each banana bite, sprinkle shredded coconut over the granola layer.

5. Drizzle with chocolate if desired: Melt the dark chocolate chips in the microwave or over a double boiler if desired. For an extra decadent touch, drizzle the melted chocolate over the banana bites.

6. Optional garnish: To add crunch and flavor, sprinkle the bits with chopped nuts.

7. Optional chilling: Refrigerate the Almond Butter Banana Bites for around 15-20 minutes to allow the almond butter to solidify somewhat.

8. Serve: Place the banana bites on a serving platter and serve.

Mango Sorbet

Ingredients:

- 4 cups ripe mango, peeled, pitted, and diced (about 4 medium-sized mangoes)
- 1/2 cup granulated sugar (adjust according to the sweetness of your mangoes)
- 1/4 cup freshly squeezed lime or lemon juice
- 1/2 cup water

Instructions

1. Mango preparation: Peel, pit, and dice the ripe mangoes until you have 4 cups total.

2. Make Easy Syrup: Combine the sugar and water in a small saucepan. Stir constantly over medium heat until the sugar is completely dissolved. Remove from the heat and set aside to cool. This results in a basic syrup.

3. Mango Blend: Combine the diced mango and lime or lemon juice in a blender or

food processor. Blend until the mixture is smooth and creamy.

4. Pour in the simple syrup: Combine the mango puree with the cooled simple syrup. Blend once more to combine.

5. Chill Blend: Refrigerate the mango mixture for at least 2 hours to allow it to cool completely.

6. Freeze: Transfer the refrigerated mixture to an ice cream maker and churn according to the manufacturer's directions. If you don't have an ice cream machine, pour the mixture into a shallow dish and freeze, stirring every 30 minutes, until it's the consistency of sorbet (approximately 4-6 hours).

7. Serve: Scoop the Mango Sorbet into individual bowls or cones.

Sweet Potato Brownies

Ingredients

- 1 cup sweet potato puree (from about 1 medium-sized sweet potato, cooked and mashed)
- 1/2 cup almond butter (or any nut or seed butter of your choice)
- 1/4 cup maple syrup or honey
- 1/4 cup unsweetened cocoa powder
- 2 tablespoons coconut flour
- 1 teaspoon vanilla extract
- 1/2 teaspoon baking powder
- A pinch of salt
- 1/2 cup dark chocolate chips (optional)
- Chopped nuts for topping (optional)

Instructions

1. Make the Sweet Potato Puree: Sweet potatoes should be cooked and mashed

until smooth. Take 1 cup of sweet potato puree.

2. Preheat the oven: Preheat the oven to 350 degrees Fahrenheit (175 degrees Celsius). Line or grease an 8x8-inch baking tray.

3. Combine the following wet ingredients: Combine the sweet potato puree, almond butter, maple syrup or honey, and vanilla extract in a large mixing bowl. Mix until everything is well blended.

4. Add the following dry ingredients: To the wet ingredients, add the cocoa powder, coconut flour, baking powder, and a bit of salt. Blend until a smooth batter is formed.

5. Optional: Toss in the chocolate chips:

6. To add richness to the brownie mixture, fold in the dark chocolate chips.

7. Transfer to a frying pan:

8. Spread the brownie batter evenly in the prepared baking sheet.

9. Bake: Bake for 20-25 minutes, or until a toothpick inserted into the center emerges with a few moist crumbs. Take care not to overbake.

10. Cool: Allow the Sweet Potato Brownies to cool for at least 10 minutes in the pan before transferring them to a wire rack to cool fully.

11. Slice: When completely cold, cut into squares or bars.

12. Optional Extras: To add crunch, put chopped nuts on top if desired.

Cherry Almond Oat Bars

Ingredients

- For the Cherry Filling:

- 2 cups fresh or frozen cherries, pitted and halved
- 1/4 cup granulated sugar
- 1 tablespoon cornstarch
- 1 tablespoon lemon juice
- For the Oat Base and Crumble:
- 1 1/2 cups old-fashioned oats
- 1 cup all-purpose flour
- 1/2 cup almond meal (ground almonds)
- 1/2 cup packed brown sugar
- 1/2 teaspoon baking soda
- 1/4 teaspoon salt
- 1/2 cup unsalted butter, melted
- 1 teaspoon almond extract
- 1/4 cup sliced almonds for topping

Instructions

1. Preheat the oven: Preheat the oven to 350 degrees Fahrenheit (175 degrees Celsius). Grease or line an 8x8-inch square baking pan.

2. Make the Cherry Filling: Combine the cherries, granulated sugar, cornstarch, and lemon juice in a medium saucepan. Cook, stirring constantly, over medium heat until the liquid thickens and the cherries release their juices. Remove from the heat and leave to cool.

3. Make the Oatmeal Base and Crumble: Combine the old-fashioned oats, all-purpose flour, almond meal, brown sugar, baking soda, and salt in a large mixing basin. Combine thoroughly.

4. Add the following wet ingredients: Melted butter and almond extract should be added now. Stir the mixture until it is uniformly blended and crumbly.

5. Assemble the Bars: To make the base of the bars, press roughly two-thirds of the oat mixture into the bottom of the prepared baking pan.

6. Spread on the Cherry Filling: Evenly distribute the chilled cherry filling over the oat foundation.

7. Finish with the remaining oat mixture: Over the cherry filling, sprinkle the leftover oat mixture. For added crunch, sprinkle with sliced almonds.

8. Bake: Bake for 25-30 minutes, or until the edges are golden brown, in a preheated oven.

9. Allow to cool before slicing: Allow the Cherry Almond Oat Bars to cool completely before cutting them into squares.

10. Serve: Serve these delectable bars with a cup of tea or coffee as a pleasant treat.

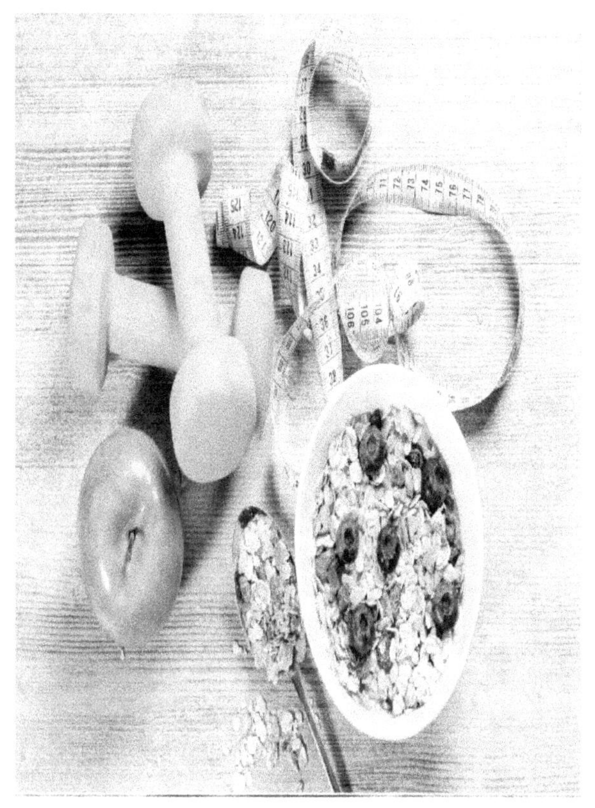

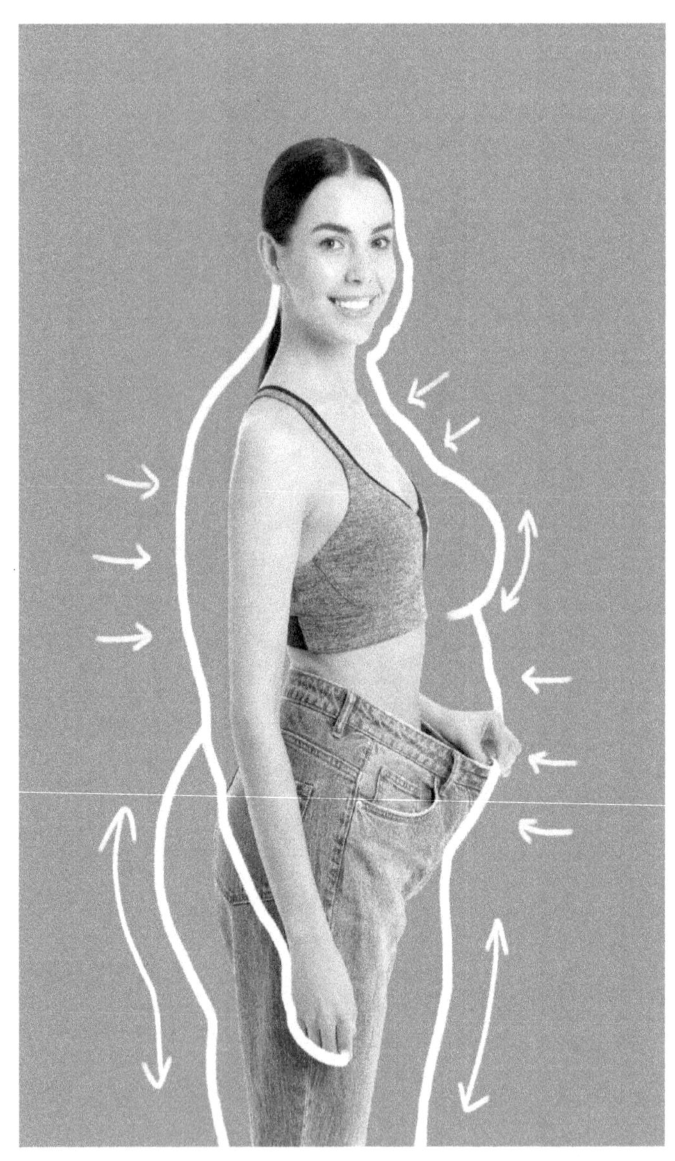

CHAPTER 6: BEVERAGES FOR WELLNESS

Green Detox Smoothie

Ingredients

- 1 cup spinach leaves, washed
- 1/2 cucumber, peeled and sliced
- 1/2 green apple, cored and chopped
- 1/2 lemon, juiced
- 1/2 inch piece of fresh ginger, peeled
- 1/2 cup pineapple chunks (fresh or frozen)
- 1/2 cup coconut water or water
- Ice cubes (optional)
- 1 tablespoon chia seeds or flaxseeds (optional, for added fiber)

Instructions

1. Prepare the following ingredients:

All of the fruits and vegetables should be washed and prepared.

2. In a blender, combine: Blend spinach leaves, cucumber slices, diced green apple, lemon juice, fresh ginger, and pineapple chunks in a blender.

3. Pour in the liquid: Fill the container halfway with coconut water or water.

4. Optional: Add the following seeds: To add fiber and nutrition, add chia seeds or flaxseeds to the blender.

5. Blend until completely smooth: Combine the ingredients in a blender until smooth and well blended. If you want a cooler smoothie, add some ice cubes to the blender.

6. Consistency should be adjusted: Add more liquid if the smoothie is too thick. If it's too thin, add a couple extra frozen pineapple chunks or ice cubes.

7. Pour and serve as follows: Fill a glass halfway with the Green Detox Smoothie.

8. Optional garnish:

9. For a decorative touch, garnish with a slice of cucumber or a wedge of lemon.

Turmeric Golden Milk

Ingredients

- 2 cups unsweetened almond milk (or any milk of your choice)
- 1 teaspoon ground turmeric
- 1/2 teaspoon ground cinnamon
- 1/4 teaspoon ground ginger
- 1 tablespoon honey or maple syrup (adjust to taste)
- 1/2 teaspoon coconut oil or ghee
- A pinch of black pepper (enhances the absorption of curcumin in turmeric)

- Optional: 1/2 teaspoon vanilla extract

Instructions

1. Prepare the following ingredients: Measure out the almond milk, turmeric powder, cinnamon powder, ginger powder, honey or maple syrup, coconut oil or ghee, and black pepper.
2. Warm the milk as follows: Warm the almond milk in a small saucepan over medium heat until it is warm but not boiling.
3. Spices to taste: To the warm milk, stir in the turmeric, cinnamon, ginger, black pepper, and coconut oil or ghee.
4. Thoroughly whisk: To incorporate the spices and make a smooth mixture, thoroughly whisk the ingredients together.

5. Simmer: Reduce the heat to low and let the mixture to simmer for 5 minutes to enable the flavors to meld.

6. Adjust the sweetness to taste: Sweeten the golden milk with honey or maple syrup according to your taste preferences. Stir well to combine.

7. Optional: Pour in the vanilla extract: Add vanilla extract for an extra layer of flavor if desired. To blend, stir everything together.

8. Optional strain: If you want the golden milk to be smoother, strain it through a fine-mesh screen to eliminate any leftover spice particles.

9. Serve: Fill mugs halfway with Turmeric Golden Milk.

Berry Bliss Smoothie

Ingredients

- 1 cup mixed berries (such as strawberries, blueberries, raspberries)
- 1 ripe banana, peeled
- 1/2 cup Greek yogurt (or non-dairy yogurt for a vegan option)
- 1/2 cup almond milk (or any milk of your choice)
- 1 tablespoon chia seeds
- 1 tablespoon honey or maple syrup (adjust to taste)
- 1/2 teaspoon vanilla extract
- Ice cubes (optional)

Instructions

1. Prepare the following ingredients: If necessary, wash the berries and hull the strawberries. Remove the peel from the ripe banana.

2. Blend in the following ingredients: Blend the mixed berries, banana, Greek yogurt, almond milk, chia seeds, honey or maple syrup, and vanilla extract in a blender.

3. Blend until completely smooth: Blend the ingredients together until they are smooth and creamy. Add ice cubes and blend again if required for a colder, thicker texture.

4. Adjust to taste: Taste the smoothie and adjust the sweetness as needed by adding more honey or maple syrup.

5. Pour into glasses as follows: Fill glasses halfway with Berry Bliss Smoothie.

6. Optional garnish: For a decorative touch, top with extra berries.

7. Serve: Enjoy this pleasant and healthful Berry Bliss Smoothie right away!

Herbal Infusion Tea

Ingredients

- 1 tablespoon dried herbal blend (such as chamomile, peppermint, lavender, or hibiscus)
- 1 teaspoon dried fruit peel (orange or lemon, for added flavor)
- 1 cinnamon stick (optional)
- 1 teaspoon honey or sweetener of choice (optional)
- 2 cups boiling water

Instructions:

1. Choose Your Herbal Blend: Depending on your preferences, select a combination of dried herbs. Chamomile for relaxing, peppermint for digestion, lavender for calming, and hibiscus for a fruity flavor are all popular options.

2. Prepare the tea infuser or tea bag: Place loose herbs in a tea infuser or tea bag for easy removal. If you don't have a tea infuser, drain the herbs once they've steeped.

3. Bring Water to a Boil: 2 cups of water should be brought to a boil. You can heat water in a kettle or on the stove.

4. Herbs in Teapot or Mug: In a teapot or directly into your mug, combine the herbal blend, dried fruit peel, and cinnamon stick (if using).

5. Boiling water should be poured: Fill the teapot or mug halfway with boiling water. Steep: Allow the herbs to infuse in the boiling water for 5 to 7 minutes. Steeping time can be varied depending on whether you desire a stronger or softer flavor.

6. (Optional): sweeten If desired, sweeten the tea with honey or your choice sweetener. To dissolve, thoroughly stir.

7. Remove or strain the infuser: If you're using loose herbs, drain the tea into a cup before removing the tea infuser or bag.

8. Serve: Fill your favorite cup or mug halfway with the Herbal Infusion Tea.

Cucumber Mint Cooler

Ingredients

- 1 large cucumber, peeled and sliced
- 1/4 cup fresh mint leaves
- 2 tablespoons honey or agave syrup (adjust to taste)
- 2 tablespoons fresh lime juice
- 2 cups cold water
- Ice cubes

- Mint sprigs and cucumber slices for garnish

Instructions

1. Cucumber and mint should be prepared as follows: Peel and cut the cucumber into rounds. Take the mint leaves off the stalks.

2. Cucumber and mint should be blended: Combine the cucumber slices, mint leaves, honey or agave syrup, and fresh lime juice in a blender.

3. Blend until completely smooth: Blend the ingredients until they form a smooth green paste.

4. Optional strain: To get a smoother texture, strain the cucumber-mint combination through a fine mesh screen or cheesecloth. This step is optional, and the cooler can be served with or without the pulp.

5. Mix with cold water: Add cold water to the combined mixture in a pitcher. To blend, stir everything together thoroughly.

6. Chill: Place the pitcher in the refrigerator for at least 30 minutes to chill.

7. Serve with ice: Fill glasses with ice cubes and pour the chilled Cucumber Mint Cooler over the ice when ready to serve.

8. Garnish: Garnish each glass with a sprig of mint and a slice of cucumber.

9. Stir and Serve: On a hot day, give it a gently swirl and enjoy this delicious Cucumber Mint Cooler!

Protein-Packed Almond Shake

Ingredients

- 1 cup unsweetened almond milk

- 1 scoop vanilla protein powder (plant-based or whey, as per your preference)
- 1 medium banana, frozen
- 2 tablespoons almond butter
- 1/2 teaspoon ground cinnamon
- 1/2 teaspoon vanilla extract
- 1 tablespoon chia seeds (optional)
- Ice cubes (optional for a colder shake)
- Honey or maple syrup to sweeten (optional)

Instructions:

1. Combine the following ingredients:
2. Blend the unsweetened almond milk, vanilla protein powder, frozen banana, almond butter, ground cinnamon, and vanilla extract in a blender.
3. Include Chia Seeds:
4. If preferred, add chia seeds to the blender for a protein, fiber, and omega-3 fatty acid boost.

5. Sweetener Optional:

6. Add honey or maple syrup to taste if you prefer a sweeter smoothie.

7. Blend until completely smooth:

8. Blend until the mixture is smooth and creamy. If you prefer a thicker shake, add more ice cubes and combine again.

9. Adjust to taste:

10. Adjust the sweetness and thickness of the drink as desired by adding more sweetener or almond milk.

11. Pour and serve as follows:

12. Fill a glass halfway with the Protein-Packed Almond Shake.

13. Garnishes are optional.

14. For extra texture, top with a dusting of cinnamon or a few almond slices.

Ingredients

- 2 cups coconut water
- 1/2 cup aloe vera juice
- 1 tablespoon fresh lemon juice
- 1 tablespoon honey or agave nectar (adjust to taste)
- 1/4 teaspoon sea salt
- Ice cubes
- Fresh mint leaves for garnish (optional)
- Slices of lemon or cucumber for garnish (optional)

Instructions

1. Prepare the following ingredients: Make sure your coconut water is cold. You can add ice cubes afterward if you don't have pre-chilled coconut water.

2. Liquids to be combined: Combine the coconut water, aloe vera juice, and fresh lemon juice in a pitcher.

3. Sweeten: Mix with the honey or agave nectar. Adjust the sweetness to suit your taste.

4. Season with sea salt: Add the sea salt and mix well. The salt replenishes electrolytes, boosting the elixir's moisturising effects.

5. Thoroughly combine: All of the ingredients should be properly mixed.

6. Optional chilling: If you want a colder drink, place the Coconut Water Hydration Elixir in the refrigerator for about 30 minutes before serving.

7. Serve with ice: In individual glasses, pour the elixir over ice cubes.

8. Optional garnish: Garnish each glass with fresh mint leaves, lemon or

cucumber slices, or both for a flavour
boost and a beautiful touch.

9. Before serving, stir: Before serving,
gently swirl the elixir to ensure that all of
the flavours are evenly dispersed.

10. Keep Hydrated: To replace electrolytes
and keep refreshed, drink this pleasant
Coconut Water Hydration Elixir as a
hydrating beverage.

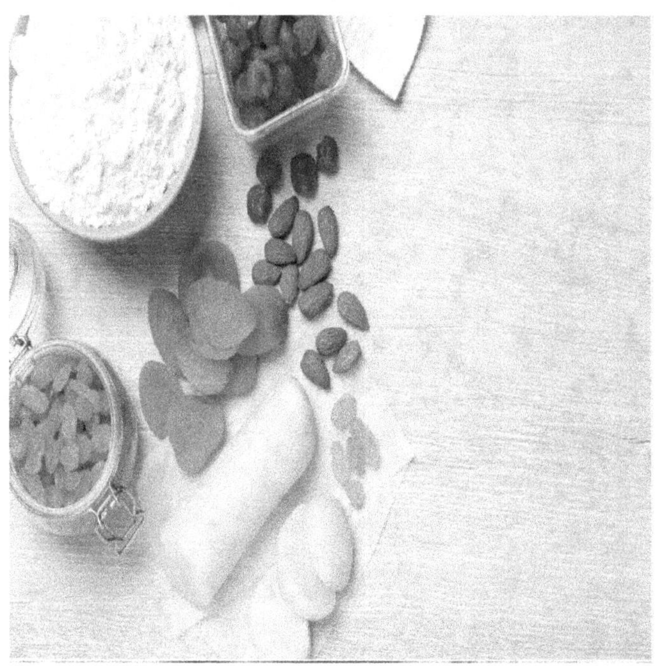

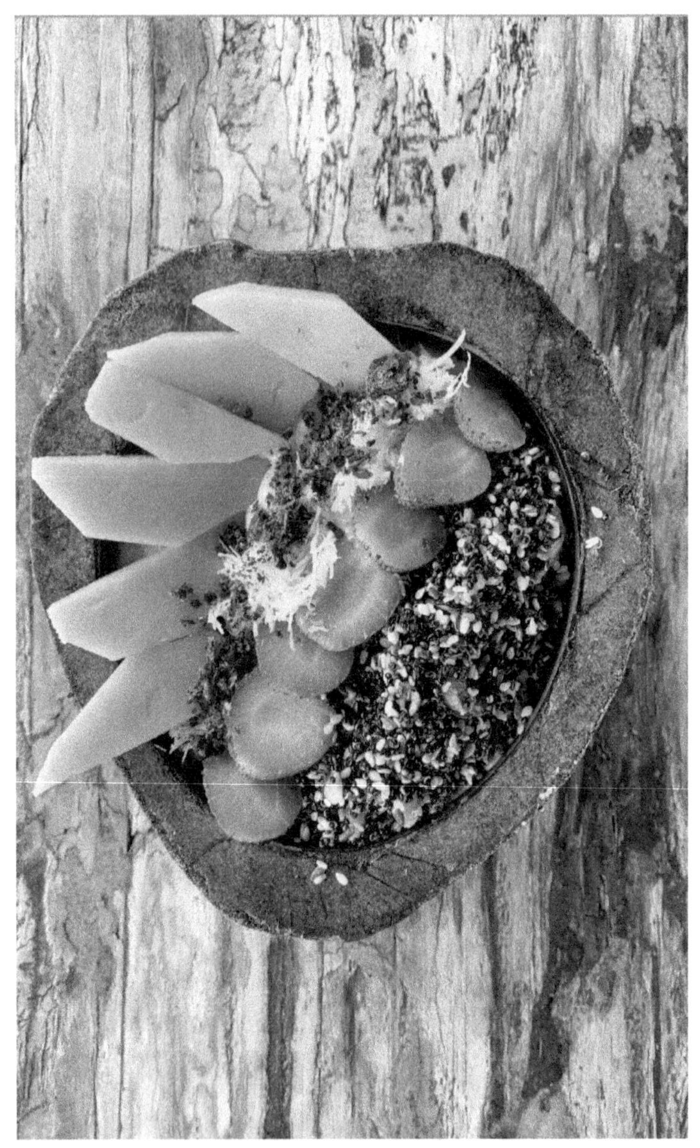

Conclusion

Additional resources:

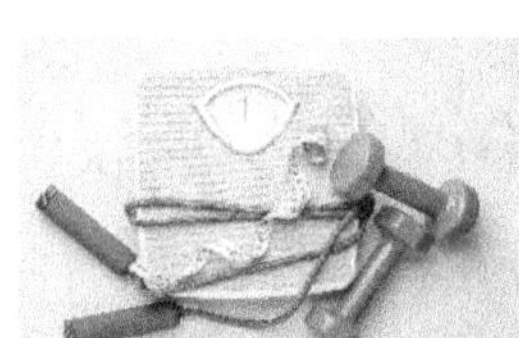

- Maintaining a healthy lifestyle becomes increasingly vital as people age. A wealth of other information are available to seniors who want to adopt a plant-based diet as part of their weight loss quest. A plant-based weight reduction cookbook suited to seniors' specific dietary needs and interests can be an important resource. Here, we look at numerous tools that may be used in conjunction with a cookbook to provide a more holistic approach to health and wellness for older people.

Nutritional and educational resources: In-depth nutritional guidelines that provide insights into important nutrients, portion control, and meal planning may be beneficial to seniors shifting to a plant-based diet. T. Colin Campbell's "The China Study" and Michael Greger's "How Not to Die" provide scientifically supported information on the benefits of a plant-based lifestyle.

culinary workshops and Workshops: Many communities and online platforms provide culinary workshops for elders. These sessions can educate seniors practical cooking skills, introduce them to new plant-based dishes, and create a safe space for them to share their experiences. Such lessons are frequently offered by local community organisations, senior centres, or online platforms such as Udemy and Skillshare.

Online Support Groups and Communities: - Joining plant-based living online communities and support groups for seniors can bring a sense of community and encouragement. Seniors can exchange recipes, discuss obstacles, and celebrate accomplishments on platforms like Facebook, Reddit, and specialist forums. Connecting with others who are on a similar path can provide motivation and develop a sense of community.

Exercise and Fitness Programs: - A well-rounded weight loss plan incorporates dietary adjustments as well as increased physical activity. Seniors might look into low-impact training programs that are appropriate for their skills and health problems. "SilverSneakers" provides individualised workout routines for older persons, supplementing the efforts of a plant-based weight control cuisine.

Holistic Health and Wellness Consultants: - Plant-based weight loss is more than simply a diet; it is a whole lifestyle shift. Stress management, sleep enhancement, and mindfulness are examples of resources that can improve the effectiveness of a weight reduction plan. Books such as Dan Buettner's "The Blue Zones" analyse the living practices of communities with outstanding lifespan and might serve as motivation for seniors.

Gardening and homegrown produce: Encouraging seniors to garden can be a satisfying addition to a plant-based diet. Growing their own fruits, veggies, and herbs guarantees not just access to fresh, organic produce, but also a pleasant and soothing outdoor activity. Gardening materials, local gardening clubs, and workshops can help seniors cultivate their own homegrown ingredients.

Routine Health Examinations and Consultation:
- Seniors should contact with healthcare specialists, such as certified dietitians or nutritionists, before making any significant dietary adjustments. Regular health check-ups can assist in tracking progress, adjusting dietary programs as needed, and ensuring that the plant-based weight loss path aligns with individual health needs.

www.ingramcontent.com/pod-product-compliance
Lightning Source LLC
Chambersburg PA
CBHW070941260726
48661CB00003B/1073